THE MAGIC
OF MELATONIN

THE MAGIC
OF MELATONIN

How This Amazing Hormone Will Help You Sleep, Reduce Pain, Relieve Anxiety, Slow Aging, and Much More

Dr. Jan-Dirk Fauteck

With the collaboration of Dr. Andrea Eder

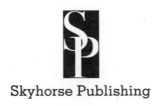

Skyhorse Publishing

This book is dedicated to you by:
Chronoceuticals, by Chronobrands

CONTENTS

Foreword   ix
Introduction   xiii

I. Fundamentals of Melatonin Research   1

Chronobiology   2
Melatonin and Its Mode of Action   24
Melatonin and the Main Fields of Application   38
Disturbances of Healthy Melatonin Production   50

II. Melatonin in Practice   55

Melatonin, the Multitalent   56
Melatonin in Various Pathologies   67
    Sleep   67
    Neuropsychiatric Disorders   85
    Headache   97
    Chronic Pain   100
    Eyes   102
    Cardiovascular Disease   106
    Digestive System   112
    Diabetes   121
    Fertility and Pregnancy   127
    Cancer   135

Summary and Outlook   144
List of Sources   147
Additional Sources   178
Picture Verification   179
About the Authors   180

FOREWORD

In this book, Dr. Fauteck summarizes critical information related to the necessity of maintaining regular biological rhythms and succinctly describes the pathological consequences of circadian rhythm disturbances—and there are many such negative side effects. One of the most fundamental and best-known rhythms is that of melatonin. Disturbance of the melatonin cycle due to any reason interferes with the sleep-wake cycle, which leads to a number of other neurobehavioral and psychological problems. It is without doubt that the consequences of the loss of melatonin and its rhythm, which normally peaks at night, far exceed sleep problems. Ample melatonin has positive effects on the brain morphology and neuronal function, as well.

Unfortunately, in modern societies, a clear distinction between day and night no longer exists because of the widespread misuse of light at night, that is, light pollution. Light at night interferes with the ability of the pineal gland to produce and disperse melatonin. As a result, either no or a severely dampened melatonin rhythm exists in individuals exposed to artificial light during the normal dark time, which includes most people living in cities and in all individuals who work at night. This suppression of a distinct melatonin rhythm and all other biological cycles represents a serious perturbation of the biological clock of many organs, contributing to pathophysiology. Chronic perturbations of biological rhythms and the melatonin cycle have been tentatively linked to a variety of neurodegenerative disorders and to an increased cancer risk. Loss of neurons is often a consequence of excessive oxidative stress that can be prevented by antioxidants. Melatonin is an uncommonly effective antioxidant, so its reduction due to the exposure to light at night may have multiple negative health consequences related to the accumulation of oxidatively damaged molecules.

In addition to the loss of melatonin resulting from the exposure to light during the normal dark period, aging usually takes a severe toll on the biological clock and on melatonin production. The reduction in the ability of humans to produce melatonin begins some time during middle age, and it is often essentially absent from the blood of elderly individuals. The drop in melatonin with aging seems to be related to many debilitating changes associated with advanced age, for example, skin deterioration, cataracts, cardiovascular disease, cancer, and neurodegeneration.

Supplemental melatonin has been widely used to correct problems of sleep disorders; its benefit in these areas stems from its ability to regulate the circadian clock. Due to its actions as a potent antioxidant, melatonin may also have benefits that protect against the ravages of aging and many age-related diseases. Dr. Fauteck comprehensively and authoritatively reviews the extensive scientific literature that illustrates the potential benefits of the use of melatonin. Melatonin is a nontoxic molecule that has been widely used by humans for many years with very few adverse events being reported. Its side effects are essentially nil.

The book by Dr. Fauteck clearly describes how melatonin is produced and secreted, how the prevailing artificially imposed light/dark cycle can disturb its rhythm, and how this translates into other potential pathologies. The author does an excellent job in explaining the relationship between disturbed circadian rhythms and suppressed melatonin levels to disease processes at a level that will be comprehensible to all readers. This is a valuable and essential contribution to understanding the association among light and darkness, the biological clock, melatonin, and human health. This book will be useful to virtually everyone who reads it. The information it contains meets a very important unmet need.

—*Russel J. Reiter, PhD, Dr. h.c. mult.*
San Antonio, Texas

INTRODUCTION

Our lives and bodies are determined by rhythms. We get up in the morning, eat several times a day, do various activities, and sleep at night. Melatonin, which is a hormone discovered only in the middle of the 1950s, is responsible for this rhythm control. Since then, it has made quantum leaps in its "career" as a subject of investigation and is a constant source of new, promising syntheses. Melatonin is known as the "Swiss army knife" (Reiter et al. 2014a) among hormones. It is a multifunctional talent with multifarious effects on our health, and it has long been a star hormone. But does it keep its promises?

Science agrees: melatonin as the multitasking hormone (Reiter et al. 2014a) has already surpassed all expectations! And there is still more to be expected, since the research is still in its infancy compared to the decades of intensive investigations of other body functions.

In addition to its sleep-aiding effect, melatonin protects our body against free radicals as a potent antioxidant and ensures a quality of life and mental fitness—even in old age. It strengthens our immune system, lowers blood pressure and cholesterol levels, and can help prevent heart disease. Recent studies also demonstrate its excellent effectiveness in the treatment of cancer, diabetes, migraine, chronic pain, eye disease, and infertility, among others. Therefore, melatonin is a true force multiplier for our health.

Imagine your organs as an orchestra that only works perfectly through a collaboration under the direction of a gifted conductor. On the conductor's desk is melatonin. Our body clock provides the rhythm and at night gives all the important body functions and organs the signal for regeneration. If our rhythm is no longer correct, our body is out of balance. This is a topic that has been the focus of chronobiology for about two decades. Thanks to this young science, we have recognized the importance of fine-tuning rhythms for our health and combating many diseases. Even now, chronobiology provides us with important physiological and pathological findings for individual medicine. However, much more is to be expected in the future of this field of study.

Melatonin is mainly produced in the pineal gland, which has been studied as "epiphysis" or "*glandula pinealis*" for thousands of years. The pinealis was first mentioned in writings by Galen of Pergamon (130–200 AD), a Greek physician and astronomer who first described its form, structure and function. Galen, as well as other Greek philosophers, saw the seat of the soul as being in the brain—especially the pinealis— and

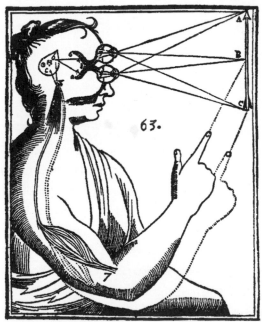

Fig. 1: Historical image by Descartes.

not in the heart, as was generally thought. (See, for example, Kunz 2006, Arendt 1995, Yu and Reiter 1992.)

René Descartes, the French philosopher and mathematician, also studied the pineal gland in search of the seat of thought. He was fascinated by the pinealis and, as a "third eye," attributed to it the control of body movements. He was convinced this was done over the eye's retina.

In the seventeenth century, this theory came to a standstill again. Scientists of this time regarded the pinealis merely as a stunted gland without any function. In the following centuries, the pine-shaped pineal gland—hence its Latin name, *glandula pinealis*—aroused the interest of research only rarely, and only half-hearted examinations were made. Nevertheless, the attempt was always made to lift its mystery, but until the middle of the last century, it kept many of its secrets.

The 1950s: Melatonin Is Discovered

Movement into modern melatonin research came in 1958 by the dermatologist Aaron Lerner. With tests on amphibians, he wanted to investigate the hormone responsible for the bleaching factor of their skin. He was particularly interested in the pineal gland, which had hitherto encountered no great scientific interest in the dermatological field. After four long years of research, Lerner was able to make the breakthrough, and he was able to name the hormone responsible for skin bleaching: "N-acetyl-5-methoxy-tryptamine," which he briefly referred to as "melatonin," a word creation from the pigment "melanin" (mela-) and the happy hormone "serotonin" (-tonin), from which melatonin is—in simplified terms—produced.

It was also Lerner who discovered the sleep-supporting effect of melatonin through a self-experiment. He took 100 mg of melatonin and noticed that, apart from great fatigue, he had no side effects. Another breakthrough came in 1963, when Richard Wurtmann found out that melatonin only enters the circulatory system in the dark.

The negative effect of light on melatonin production was first demonstrated by Alfred Lewy in 1981—an important finding also for chronobiology. Thus, it could be shown that the light-dark clock in our body is translated into a signal, which then determines our rhythm. Many contemporary researchers are especially interested in the study of this difference between day and night rhythm (e.g., jet lag) and its effects on our body and health (see also Johnston and Skene 2015).

From Hype to Intensive Research

From the 1980s onward, interest in the manifold effects of melatonin and its exploration intensified—and continues to this day (Varoni et al. 2016). Although much remains to be explored about the mode of action, studies so far suggest an even broader range of positive effects on our organism than previously assumed.

Melatonin experienced its hype in the 1990s, especially in the USA. Because it was lauded as a miracle drug, many Americans fell for the marketing ploys in books such as *The Melatonin Miracle: Nature's Age-Reversing, Disease-Fighting, Sex-Enhancing Hormone* by Walter Pierpaoli (1995). However, in *Melatonin: Breakthrough Discoveries That Can Help You Combat Aging, Boost Your Immune System, Reduce Your Risk of Cancer and Heart Disease, Get a Better Night's Sleep*, the studies and tests all rejected the miraculous promises of the *Melatonin Miracle* publication; skepticism about the ambiguous and hoped-for effect of melatonin was the result (Reiter and Robinson 1995).

In the following decades, interest in melatonin developed dramatically. In 1995, 465 studies on melatonin were published, according to PubMed, an English-language database with scientific articles on overall biomedicine. In 2016, there were 1,092 papers published in highly scientific journals. As you can see, research interest in melatonin has grown enormously. A total of 21,893 reviews are currently published on PubMed (as of January 2017) that deal with the effects of melatonin.

I. FUNDAMENTALS OF MELATONIN RESEARCH

Chronobiology

Chronobiology, the science of inner rhythms, is derived from the Greek words "chrónos" (time), "bíos" (life), and "logos" (word). It describes our biological rhythms that are influenced by internal (endogenous) and external (exogenous) clocks, which influence each other. Heartbeat, breathing, sleep—all these are controlled by our inner rhythms.

The most important exogenous clock is the sun. Before ancient times, when our ancestors had not even discovered fire for themselves, man adapted himself to this natural timer. One worked from dawn to dusk; nighttime was the impetus for sleep and regeneration.

The Rhythm of Our Body

Hormones, organs, our whole body follow a certain rhythm, which is subsequently subjected to the time of day. Have you ever bought shoes early in the morning? How did you feel when you tried your new purchase in the evening to go out? Did they fit as well as at the beginning of the day? Probably not, and that is related to your feet swelling later in the day, in turn with the rhythm of your body.

Or another example: When do you prefer to cuddle with your partner? Probably in the evening, and this is completely normal. Science has long known that sex hormones are not at their peak before going to sleep, but rather in the morning, when the sexual organs are well perfused and soft. On the other hand, the so-called cuddle hormone has its climax in the evening.

As you can see, all the processes in our bodies are determined by a rhythm that is sometimes measurable, as the shoe example shows. Like our feet, our body size also varies between

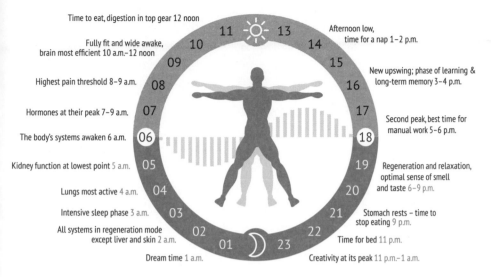

Time to eat, digestion in top gear 12 noon

Fully fit and wide awake,
brain most efficient 10 a.m.–12 noon

Highest pain threshold 8–9 a.m.

Hormones at their peak 7–9 a.m.

The body's systems awaken 6 a.m.

Kidney function at lowest point 5 a.m.

Lungs most active 4 a.m.

Intensive sleep phase 3 a.m.

All systems in regeneration mode
except liver and skin 2 a.m.

Dream time 1 a.m.

Afternoon low,
time for a nap 1–2 p.m.

New upswing; phase of learning &
long-term memory 3–4 p.m.

Second peak, best time for
manual work 5–6 p.m.

Regeneration and relaxation,
optimal sense of smell
and taste 6–9 p.m.

Stomach rests – time to
stop eating 9 p.m.

Time for bed 11 p.m.

Creativity at its peak 11 p.m.–1 a.m.

Fig. 2: The rhythm of life.

one and two centimeters in the course of a day. For medical diagnostics, it is also important to observe the laws of chronobiology: a blood analysis taken in the evening shows more blood corpuscles than in the morning.

Unconsciously, you are already applying the regularities of chronobiology: If you are a woman, you may wear a lighter skin cream with UV protection in the morning than in the evening. If you are on a diet, you probably do not have a calorie bomb in the evening. Many people refrain from coffee after a certain time, because they then find it very difficult to fall asleep. Chronobiology thus determines many of our daily actions without consciously perceiving them. (See Fig. 2.)

Chronobiology: Previously Smiled Upon, Recognized Today

Chronobiology did not establish itself as an independent scientific discipline until the mid-to-late 1980s. Only from this point onward were the daily rhythmic fluctuations of our body (for example, heart rate, blood pressure, or body temperature) no longer regarded as pathological phenomena, but as physiological, natural processes.

What had been smiled upon three decades before is intensively explored today—with impressive and amazing results on the interplay of body, mind, and time. Research has shown that heart rate, blood pressure, and body temperature fluctuate rhythmically during the day. For example, your body temperature is higher in the morning than in the evening. This is a completely natural process, because your body adapts to its surroundings.

If this adaptation is absent or your biotic rhythms are interfered with, the result is stress on the organism—often with serious consequences for your health. Think of people who do shift work every day, with completely different day-night rhythms. Studies have shown that they suffer much more frequently from diabetes, hypertension, and cancer. Their inner rhythms are completely out of balance, actually working against their rhythm, which can lead to problems with digestion, nervousness, sleep disorders, heart disease, reduced memory, and reduced concentration. All these rhythmic disturbances have one thing in common: an interrupted, often reduced, melatonin production.

The choked melatonin production also disrupts processes of cell division and repair, which increases the risk of tumor formation. Older (e.g., Reiter and Robinson 1995) and recent (e.g., Vetter et al. 2016, Bhatti et al. 2016, Qian and Scheer 2016) studies always conclude that every disturbance of our natural rhythm or altered release of melatonin has serious consequences on our health.

The Third Eye: Melatonin as an Ambassador of the Day-Night Rhythm

Light and darkness—these phenomena determine our wakefulness and our sleep—in short, our day-night rhythm. Melatonin, the hormone of the dark, transmits the information "nighttime" to our brain and all other organs in our body:

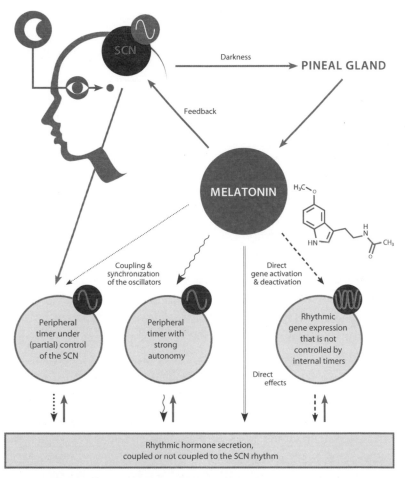

Fig. 3: Schematic representation of the complex linking of different timers (modified by Hardeland 2013).

The body temperature drops, and our organs begin with their regeneration.

Melatonin is mainly formed in the pineal gland (the so-called "third eye"). It has this name because every light pulse is passed from the retina of the eye to the internal clock, the SCN—suprachiasmatic nucleus—which is a switching center of our brain. The SCN, in turn, is connected to the pineal gland by a complex route, where the melatonin is formed mainly at night in complete darkness.

Other places in the body where melatonin is produced during the day are the digestive tract, blood platelets, retina, testes or ovaries, spinal cord, lymphocytes, and skin. The melatonin that is also produced in daylight has especially local effects, for example, in its effect as an antioxidant. To what extent and whether the melatonin produced here affects the melatonin production in the pineal gland at night, and thus also functions as a superimposed timer, is still the subject of investigations. (See Fig. 3.)

Biological Rhythms: Transmitted Light and Darkness

Melatonin is produced in and released from the pineal gland, especially in the dark. Light, however, suppresses this production. The information "darkness" is passed on by melatonin to almost all cells and organs. The hormone acts as an internal signal and time generator for the cells and organs, because each cell follows a certain rhythm. (See Fig. 4.)

During the day, very little melatonin is produced, and intensive production begins only in the evening. At around 11 p.m., the "sleep" level rises to eight times the daily rate. This is the signal for the command "night operation" to the organs, and the brain then stores important information from the day to long-term memory.

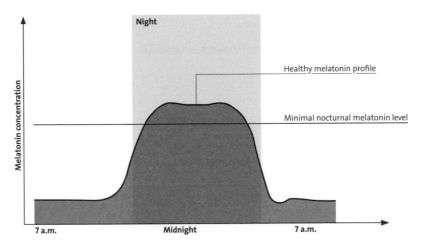

Fig. 4: Schematic representation of the normal melatonin rhythm of an adult.

These rest periods are life-giving and health-promoting for our bodies. This is also shown by the fact that today's science distinguishes more than one hundred maladies that are regarded as sleep-related! (See Fig. 5.)

Our sleep can be disturbed by a number of causes. We live in a time when we are constantly exposed to light: the TV and mobile phone with their blue lights, the alarm clock next to our beds—all of these devices are rhythm destroyers, which disrupt our melatonin production (e.g., Chang et al. 2015).

On the other hand, studies have shown that red light significantly and positively affects nightly melatonin production and can even help people with a sleep disorder (delayed phase sleep disorder or DPSD) get a healthy night's sleep (Esaki et al. 2016).

On our external retina, sensory cells ensure that we perceive the difference between light and dark. This information is transmitted to the brain via the so-called photoreceptors via the nerve cells, and then to the pineal gland, followed by all the organs in our bodies.

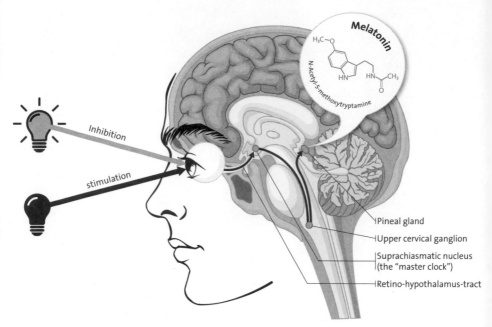

Fig. 5: Complex neural linkage of the eye with the pineal gland. As soon as light falls on the retina, the production of melatonin in the pineal organ is blocked.

What Are Photoreceptors?

Photoreceptors are cells that contain a high amount of the pigment melanopsin and that react particularly to light. Besides the rods and cones in the human eye, they are important for light reception.

Even blind people, if their retina is not completely destroyed, perceive the difference between darkness and light. It is only a sensation of light that is often not consciously perceived. Nonetheless, visually impaired people usually have more sensitive photoreceptors, which react very sensitively to every slight change in light. This is also one reason why depression (seasonal affective disorder, or SAD), a condition that is linked to, among other things, disturbed melatonin production, affects them three times as often (Madsen et al. 2016a).

But what is biological rhythm? The question cannot be answered unequivocally, since our chronobiology knows many rhythms of different lengths. Our bodies produce some, and others are determined by external environmental influences. One thing is certain: every regular biological process automatically creates its own biological rhythm. In turn, almost all rhythms are interrelated, so that they interact with and regulate one another. The day-night rhythm and the resulting melatonin rhythm play a major role by synchronizing many of the body's rhythms.

The most important rhythms can be described in regard to their respective period (e.g., by the time they need to cycle through, or by what influences them).

Circadian Rhythms

A circadian rhythm is a biological rhythm with a periodic duration of approximately twenty-four hours. Body temperature, the production of many hormones, pain sensitivity and performance, motor activity, and many other important processes are controlled by circadian rhythms.

The most important circadian rhythm for humans is the sleep-wake rhythm. Light is the strongest external clock of the circadian system, as it influences the timing of many physiological processes, including the daily variation of melatonin production. Incidentally, melatonin is detectable not only in the blood, but in almost every body fluid and is the hormone with the greatest concentration of fluctuations within twenty-four hours.

Ultradian and Infradian Rhythms

If a rhythm has a duration of fewer than twenty-four hours, one speaks of an ultradian rhythm; more than twenty-four hours is an infradian rhythm. Do you feel hungry at regular intervals? The ultradian rhythm is responsible for this. On the other hand, bowel movements and sexuality are controlled by the infradian rhythm. Nature also knows its rhythms. For example, the ebb and flow of the tides follow the ultradian rhythm.

In a study, a link between ultradian rhythms and mental health was established (Blum et al. 2014). Our sensation of hunger follows an ultradian rhythm of about four hours, which seems to be regulated primarily by dopamine, a neurotransmitter. Since dopamine plays a central role in mental health, dopamine imbalance has consequences for our mental health. Disorders of the dopamine level have been discovered in various mental illnesses, from schizophrenia to bipolar disorders. Recent studies have shown that disturbances of circadian rhythms (e.g., the release of melatonin) can adversely affect these ultradian rhythms (Tosini et al. 2008) and thus can cause both eating and memory disorders.

Circannual Rhythms

The circannual rhythm has a duration of roughly one year. The seasons with their effects on our minds or our immune systems are examples of how this temporal rhythm affects our conditions. Do you have a greater need for sleep or greater appetite for noodles, potatoes, and other starchy foods in the winter months? Then you can thank your circannual rhythm, which affects up to 25 percent of all people. Especially in this group of people, the prolonged melatonin distribution during the winter months seems to influence other rhythms.

There are also other rhythms, such as the septennial rhythm, marked by the algal blooms every seven years. If you are planning your next holiday, make sure you know when your holiday destination has been flooded with algae for the last time. On the other hand, a typical circalunar rhythm is the menstrual cycle of the woman, which is repeated every twenty-eight days.

Endogenous and Exogenous Rhythms

All the rhythms that our body produces itself are called endogenous rhythms, including, for example, the heart or respiratory rate, or the rhythmic hormone release. The endogenous rhythm remains largely the same, even if our environmental conditions change. On the other hand, exogenous rhythms, which are controlled by environmental influences, act on us from the outside (e.g., the day-night change or food intake).

Endogenous and exogenous rhythms usually influence each other. For example, cool temperatures in the morning make us wake up, no matter how deep the sleep. However, there are also rhythms that are largely independent of one another, such as renal function, which is relatively self-sufficient, or the release of insulin. Regardless of food intake, the pancreas pours out insulin three times a day: morning, noon, and evening. But the most important pulse generator in our body—melatonin—can synchronize all rhythms.

The Inner Clocks: The Orchestra of All Organs

Everyone has different internal clocks that influence one another. The hormones in our bodies also follow a rhythm. They are timed, such as sex hormones for reproduction, stress hormones for disease suppression, and control hormones that regulate our eating habits.

Our body's rhythms are based on a "main clock" and many "secondary clocks." The main clock, the SCN (suprachiasmatic nucleus), sits in the brain. Imagine an atomic clock for all digital clocks.

This function is executed by the SCN. In turn, this rhythm is determined daily by the change of brightness and darkness, that is, day and night, and is adjusted every day to the twenty-four-hour rhythm. (See Fig. 6.)

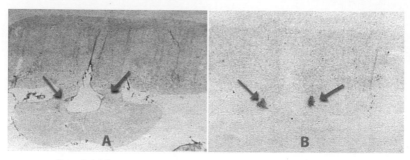

Fig. 6A: Melatonin receptors on the human internal clock (SCN).
Microscopic representation of the hypothalamus region with the seat of the SCN.
Fig. 6B: Melatonin receptors in the SCN.

The SCN provides the circadian rhythm and transmits it via the nervous system and the hormones to the other organs. The adjoining clocks are thus aligned with the main clock. If this complex interplay of watches is permanently disrupted—called chronodisruption—this can lead to numerous illnesses.

Besides melatonin, the hormone cortisol (produced in the adrenal gland) plays a key role in our circadian rhythm. Between 4 and 5 a.m., it rises continually, reaching its peak at 8:30 a.m. As the day progresses, cortisol levels drop until they reach their lowest level at midnight, then reenter their circulation four or five hours later.

Our central "main clock," the SCN, and the peripheral "auxiliary clocks" also seem to be controlled and synchronized by cortisol, and they control our day-clock rhythm. Because melatonin makes us sleep in the night, cortisol gets us up in the morning and takes care of our activity during the day until the evening, when it hands over the scepter to the hormone of the dark. It is interesting to note that a shift of the melatonin rhythm almost always causes a shift in cortisol release.

From the Lark to the Night Owl and Back Again

All people are different. This sentence also applies to our internal clocks, because not all people live the same rhythm. And this is not enough; our rhythm changes several times over a lifetime.

Are you an early bird or a night owl? Or has it changed in the course of your life? Do you have children going through puberty? Then you know how hard it is to get them out of bed in the morning and how they like to make the night a day. On the other hand, older people often complain that they get up with the chickens and are ready for bed before the evening film. These examples show that our age influences our inner clock and thus also our sleep-wake rhythm.

But apart from whether you are a young adult and can dance the night away at parties or rather admire the sunrise in the morning, people are as individual as their optimal daytime activities. Healthy mix types of night owl and those who prefer morning are quite common and completely natural if not the rule (see test 1, pp. 15–18).

But why do older people often complain about insomnia and are generally less likely to sleep than people who are still growing up? The answer is simple: in the elderly, the melatonin level is significantly lower, and the nightly release takes place for significantly fewer hours than in children, adolescents, or younger adults. Studies have shown that more than 80 percent of all elderly people have a melatonin deficiency! This is also the reason why older people often suffer from sleep disorders, which in turn leads to the conclusion that the so-called senile flight from bed does not exist! The causes of intermittent or early waking problems are, rather, due to diminished melatonin production. Some figures for a better understanding: melatonin is highest at the age of one to three years. At the age of seventy, the melatonin level is often less than one-tenth of this peak, and the duration of the secretion is no longer six to seven hours, but rather only two to three hours (Yonei et al. 2010). (See Fig. 7.)

The American sleep medic Michael Breus speaks of four chronotypes: bear, dolphin, lion, and wolf. Yet they overlap with the lark, the owl, and the mixed type (Breus 2016).

The melatonin production of the body goes through many changes throughout our lives. Even the unborn child in the mother's body has melatonin receptors but cannot produce melatonin on its own and is dependent on the mother. Babies up to their first year of life do not yet have a marked day-night rhythm, which is clocked by the melatonin, and thus only wake up during eating times.

From the first year of life, melatonin production rises to a very high level, reaches its highest values in the third year

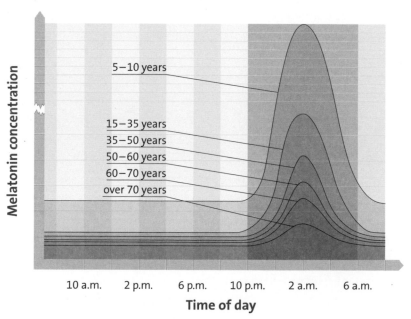

Fig. 7: Age-dependent change in melatonin level.

of life, and continues into puberty. Children also have to cope with disturbances in their melatonin production due to, for example, a night-light, noise, or social stress factors.

When puberty is reached, this high melatonin level is dramatically reduced. You can imagine it like a house of cards, which collapses in one fell swoop. It is precisely this melatonin fracture that initiates puberty! Young people are classic "owls" who like to sleep long and do not get to bed in the evening. The distribution of melatonin is delayed in the case of adolescents, which is the reason for the feeling of fatigue late in the day, as studies always show (Crowley et al. 2016).

These "symptoms" decrease with age, so that most adults from the age of twenty return to a normal rhythm. Yet the pineal gland also loses its ability to produce melatonin in adequate amounts over time. One reason for this is presumed to be the reduced blood circulation of this organ, which is exacerbated by the intake of certain medicines or too much alcohol. If there is also stress in everyday life or light during the night, melatonin production is even more suppressed.

Test 1: What Chronotype Are You: Night Owl, Lark, or Intermediate?

> I don't mind getting up early in the morning at all.
Ⓐ True   Ⓑ Not true at all

> In the evening, I go to bed between 9 and 10 p.m.
Ⓐ True   Ⓑ Not true at all

> In the evening, I read for at least a half hour before falling asleep.
Ⓐ True   Ⓑ Not true at all

> In the evening, I like to drink one or more glasses of wine or beer.
Ⓐ True   Ⓑ Not true at all

❭ I sleep much longer in the morning on holidays.
Ⓐ True   Ⓑ Not true at all

❭ I love to meet up with friends in the evening.
Ⓐ True   Ⓑ Not true at all

❭ If there were no household work, I would go to bed earlier in the evening.
Ⓐ True   Ⓑ Not true at all

❭ You cannot get me out of bed before 7 a.m., even on a weekday.
Ⓐ True   Ⓑ Not true at all

❭ I use my weekends to finally catch up on sleep.
Ⓐ True   Ⓑ Not true at all

❭ I wake up feeling rested five out of seven days.
Ⓐ True   Ⓑ Not true at all

❭ Most of the time, I wake up at the right time by myself.
Ⓐ True   Ⓑ Not true at all

❭ I work most efficiently in the morning.
Ⓐ True   Ⓑ Not true at all

❭ On New Year's Eve, I plan a nap during the day.
Ⓐ True   Ⓑ Not true at all

Test Evaluation: What Chronotype Are You?

Adults seem to have two phases of sleep in sleep-medical research. On the one hand, the first four hours are the so-called vital sleeping phase. This sleeping phase is an absolute must for regeneration and recovery and the processing of the most important experiences of the day. All additional hours of sleep are what are referred to as optional sleep in adults. It also serves to keep the organism healthy and to process the results of the day. However, its temporal extent and its availability are not indispensable. The exhaustion of this optional sleep seems to mark a great difference in the subjective feeling between the two sleeping types designated as night owl and lark.

The differences in the metabolic parameters observed in a recent study between the night owl and lark—in the sense that late bedtimes are connected not only to a tendency to have higher body mass index as well as abdominal circumference, but also to higher blood lipid values and insulin levels in the morning—can be based on two factors. On the one hand, energy consumption is higher in the waking state than in sleep. This lowers the sugar level and directly stimulates sugar regeneration. On the other hand, this can lead to late additional food intake. Also, in that case, development toward increasing blood pressure, for example, is guaranteed.

The type one belongs to has no influence on the composition of meals. Only the time when the appropriate meals should ideally be taken changes: the lark is slightly earlier than the owl, with the breaks between meals remaining the same.

If the body misses breakfast, which is earlier for the lark than for the night owl, the risk of insulin secretion stimulation increases. And also for the late risers who eat breakfast around noon, one should be going easy on the insulin stimulation.

Overall Results

More "A" Replies: Lark

With your answers, you have given mostly indications that your sleep type is a convincing lark. Your performance peak is in the early morning or later in the morning. You have a relatively easy time getting up early in the morning, are tired in the evening, and are happy when you can go to sleep when your body tells you to. You can optimize your sleep hygiene by having dinner early in the evening and also in a family environment. Promote peace and quiet at home from a relatively early hour, for example, 9 p.m., so that you can follow your rhythm.

More "B" Replies: Night Owl

With your answers, you have mostly indicated that you are the typical night owl, also known as an owl. Getting up early is a horror for you. In the evening, you can amp up again, but during the week you also need your time to calm down and go to bed in time to be able to cope with the pressures of everyday life. As your food intake times also move backward on the time axis of the day, you should—especially with your profession and professional commitments—ensure that your sleeping habits are as optimal as possible. This means, in concrete terms, the exploitation of the latest start of work at a flexible time and a profession in which you have to start your day at a later hour. If possible, begin work in the afternoon and work into the evening hours—that should be an ideal schedule for you.

The Same Amount of "A" and "B" Answers

You are more or less in the middle with your answers and have the same arguments for both sides. Obviously, you belong to the majority of people, who are called mixed types. It is advisable for you to always go back and listen to yourself in order to find out in which direction your body points you. More night owl? More lark? Try to optimize your sleep hygiene according to the basic determination of your tendency.

Environmental Influences

Around one-third of our lives is spent sleeping, which is an important time in which our bodies and their organs can regenerate. Our brain also needs this resting phase to sort, process, and store information in the long-term memory.

Do you have an easy time sleeping, getting a good night's rest, and thus feel refreshed in the morning? Congratulations!

But how do you manage to change from summer to winter, and vice versa? Or how do you deal with jet lag?

Any change in the environment has an impact on our bodies. Sometimes we can adjust in advance, but only if these changes happen regularly. For example, this is the case when changing from day to night. We can also adapt to alternating phases of activity and recovery. One speaks in these cases of adaptation or temporal synchronization.

Watch yourself when the next winter or summer comes: Do you have more need for sleep or do you wake up almost automatically in the morning as soon as the first rays of sun fall into your bedroom? In the warm months of the year, what do you have more appetite for: a crispy, refreshing salad or a warming stew that will make you feel nice and full? (See Fig. 8.)

Our body adapts to the seasons—almost unnoticeably for you. Of course, these adjustments or synchronizations also affect all biochemical processes in our bodies. And that's good. This adaptation is also possible because the respective changes of the seasons are creeping by slowly. The body has enough time to adjust. For example, if these adjustments are not made because there is not enough time between changes, this has serious consequences for our health and well-being. One then speaks of an abrupt disturbance of the inner rhythm or of an "acute chronodisruption." Man lives according to his inner clock.

For example, most accidents happen between 2 and 3 a.m., regardless of whether people are well rested or not! An Italian study examined the melatonin level of hospital workers to determine whether there is a link between the risk of injury and a low level of melatonin. The study confirmed that subjects who had not been injured had higher melatonin levels than those who had been injured (Valent et al. 2016). The subjects

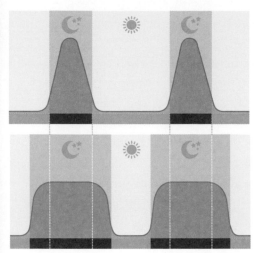

Summer
long days
short melatonin signal

Duration of melatonin synthesis as a function of the season

Winter
short days
long melatonin signal

Fig. 8: Duration of melatonin synthesis as a function of day length/season
(modified by Arendt 1995).

who had less melatonin performed shift work and had not yet gotten used to the new rhythm.

Also, the change to daylight savings time—with one hour more of sunlight, but also an hour less of sleep—can have serious consequences. Shortly after the time change, an 8 percent increase in having a stroke was observed. Although this value normalized after a few days, the study shows that even this slight shift of the day-night rhythm has a serious effect on our bodies because the body needs time to adjust (Sipilä et al. 2016).

Differences between the Sexes

Another study has shown that men and women react differently to the repeated alteration of their day-night rhythm. Both sexes showed great fatigue symptoms, but women showed a diminished performance in cognitive and memory tests, especially in the early morning hours. It is assumed that various factors are responsible for this. In addition to hormonal causes, it seems that women simply need more sleep, which is due to the increased activities in their daily lives. Further research is required in order to be able to design better treatments or preventive measures (Santhi et al. 2016).

Readjust the Internal Clock with Light and Melatonin Therapy

Scientists have long been concerned with the question of how to treat and deal with the many symptoms of shift workers. The solution sounds simple, but it is in the details and in the right timing. With chronotherapy, the internal clock can be tricked.

Certain sources of light have proved to be a good way to shift the nocturnal melatonin production toward the day. Specific melatonin preparations, especially in combination with light therapy, are also recommended. The aim of this therapy is to produce a new melatonin twenty-four-hour rhythm, which is synchronized with the new active/rest rhythm, even if it does not correspond to the actual day-night rhythm.

Environmental Light

How do you feel after a long day working at the office, where you have not experienced any direct sunshine? Or, imagine it is November and there is a foggy grayness dominating the days. The sun seems to be swallowed up by the ground. How do you feel? Are you in a good, upbeat mood?

Most people will say no to this last question and will rather describe the "bad and clouded mood" that they experience. And that's quite natural. Because light and the sun have been proven to be pick-me-ups and true lucky charms, people who are regularly in natural surroundings, thus exposing themselves to daylight, demonstrate fewer depressive moods, less fatigue, or ravenous appetites. Try it!

On the contrary, the artificial light in the evening, which we can barely escape, is detrimental to our rhythm. Melatonin production is suppressed and, if necessary, shifted. In this case, we speak of "social jet lag," a condition we have created by the effects of electric environmental lighting. Its impact on our body is comparable to jet lag after overseas flights.

In addition, the symbiosis of serotonin and melatonin is responsible for the negative effects of jet lag and shift work: they belong together as day and night or light and dark. While the serotonin during the day ensures that you are lively and full of energy, the melatonin in the evening creates the peace that you need to rejuvinate your body. The perfect interplay of this duo is the guarantee for your health.

Our modern lifestyle, however, often throws the two out of balance. We spend the whole day in artificial light instead of natural sunlight; in the evening, we sleep in front of the TV or read the latest headlines of the day in the bed on our smartphones or tablets. Also, the streetlights illuminating our rooms from the outside are difficult to switch off. "Social jet lag" is thus preprogrammed.

In the Evening: Lights Off

Not only does too little sunshine or bright light interrupt our biorhythms, but too little darkness delays the production of melatonin and thus our sleep, which leads to chronodisruption and eliminates our circadian rhythm. Studies show a connection among diabetes, fatigue, heart disease, and some tumor diseases (e.g., Michael et al. 2015).

A study investigated the effect of so-called blue light on mobile phones or computers. While it does not show any negative effects on our body during the day, it seems to be very negative to our rhythm during the night, as it inhibits the formation of melatonin and affects our sleep. The problem of nocturnal blue light has been increasing since energy-efficient LEDs have become widely used in modern technology. We hope, in the near future, new lamps will be introduced that do not block melatonin production. Initial investigations show that light with other wavelengths (e.g., red light) influenced the melatonin production less strongly (Bonmati-Carrion et al. 2014).

If you have children, you probably know their fear of the dark. A bedside lamp or the like is then switched on in the nursery so that the little ones can fall asleep quietly. In this case, please remember to switch off the light or to equip it with a timer. A permanent source of light damages sleep and thus the health of your child. If you cannot or do not want to do without light, for your child's sake, use red light.

Melatonin and Its Mode of Action

Although we have known of the hormone melatonin since 1958, it took a long time to find out how exactly it is produced and broken down in the body and how it works.

Synthesis and Metabolism

The trio of melatonin, serotonin, and tryptophan controls important biosynthetic processes in our body and interacts with one another. Serotonin, the body's happy hormone, is formed from the amino acid tryptophan and is further transformed into melatonin during the night.

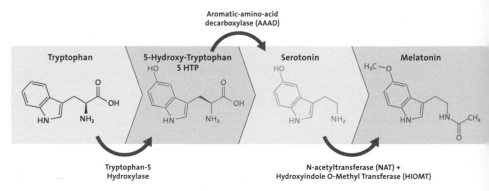

Fig. 9: Structural formulas of the substances from which melatonin is produced.

Serotonin: The Happiness Hormone

While melatonin regulates our day-night rhythm and is mainly released during the night, serotonin is produced mainly during the day, especially in the morning. It improves our mood and increases our drive. In the short term, serotonin can also be increased via carbohydrates and sugars; you know the comfort you feel when you have eaten a portion of pasta or chocolate. In this case, insulin is released in the body, which, in addition to the sugar utilization in our body, also increases the uptake of the protein building block tryptophan into the brain. And then a new interaction begins: tryptophan is converted into serotonin, and your mood improves.

The mood is not only improved by chocolate or a serotonin-rich banana, but also by physical exercise. Serotonin is also released during physical activity, in addition to many other hormones that have a positive effect on your health.

Serotonin acts as a messenger for some of our most important body functions, such as the regeneration of the liver and pancreas, or blood coagulation, as well as our gastrointestinal activity. For example, serotonin also controls the tension of our vessels and thus affects a migraine or heart problems.

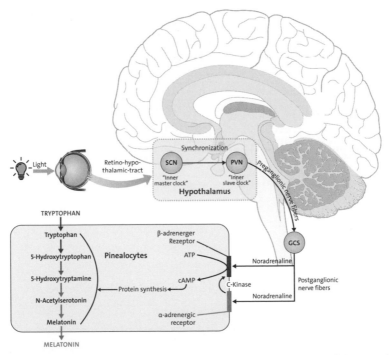

Fig. 10: Complex control loop, in which factors block the function of the pineal gland (modified according to Arendt 1995).

Serotonin Deficiency

A serotonin deficiency is very often responsible for sleep disorders, depression, impotence, fatigue, and even breathing problems.

The lack of light during the winter months can be a cause of a deficiency, as well as a lack of hormones and vitamins, chronic stress, emotional extremes, inflammation in the body, and so forth. Many studies show that a relationship exists between serotonin deficiency and seasonal depression, or SAD (e.g., McMahon et al. 2016).

If too little serotonin is produced, a snowball effect is established. In particular, melatonin is no longer produced in the body to a sufficient degree. Since serotonin is the main precursor for melatonin production in the evening, it is also possible to explain why serotonin deficiency can lead to insomnia.

Numerous studies are continually investigating the interrelationships of melatonin and serotonin (e.g., Kamal et al. 2015), with great prospects for the treatment of mental disorders or chronic pain. The importance of the aforementioned symbiosis of this duo, as well as possible disturbances of its rhythm, is becoming increasingly recognized.

Cellular Effects of Melatonin

Melatonin acts in the body through many different mechanisms. Some of them function by means of so-called receptors, which sit either on the cell membrane or inside the cell, while others act without these docking sites.

The receptors that are membrane-bound include the melatonin receptor MTL1 (also Mel1a) and MTL2 (also Mel1b). Both belong to the family of transmembrane receptors, which are coupled to G proteins and on whose exterior surface melatonin can dock. When this occurs, different biochemical processes occur within the cell, which then also lead to the effect of melatonin in those cells (see, e.g., Jockers et al. 2008, Emet et al. 2016).

Imagine a door lock that can only be opened from the outside. Melatonin is the key with which you can enter. This process can, for example, trigger the release of enzymes or calcium, thus initiating important processes for our body.

A third receptor called MRR, or GPR50, within the cell is still very little researched and is probably not very important for humans, unlike certain animal species. The exact function of these receptors is the subject of ongoing investigations (Jockers et al. 2016).

Different Receptor Distributions in Humans and Animals

There are marked differences in the receptor distribution between different animal species and humans. Animals such as rodents and most mammals have receptors especially in those areas that control their internal clock and gonad function—organs used for the production of sexual hormones and offspring. This is mainly due to the fact that these animals only reproduce at certain times of the year. Unlike us humans, who are not seasonally limited in our fertility and our ability to reproduce.

The chronobiologist Jürgen Aschoff made one of the first investigations (Aschoff and Meyer-Lohmann 1955): by adding melatonin to their food, he transitioned male hamsters to a schedule with a darkness lasting more than twelve hours and thus to an artificial winter phase. As a result, their testicles shrank, and they were no longer able to reproduce. This condition lasted six to eight weeks, then the hamsters noticed that they were being misled, and their testicles formed sperm again.

Most species do not have receptors in the cerebral cortex and almost none in the cerebellar cortex. This is quite different from humans, who have the most receptors in the cerebellum, in the cerebral cortex, and in the pineal glands. In those areas that are responsible for reproduction, humans have virtually no receptors. For example, the melatonin action via the melatonin receptors in the cerebellar cortex thus provides signals so that we completely relax our muscles while we sleep. However, an animal does not know any complete muscle relaxation and is always ready to flee—even in sleep.

In addition to the cerebrum, the human body has many other areas in the body where melatonin receptors can be found. They are distributed throughout the body's organs and cell structures, such as the spinal cord, retina, spleen, pituitary gland, liver, kidney, thymus, heart, and lungs, and less so in the testicles, pancreas, lymphocytes, and blood vessels. Melatonin receptors have also been found in the uterus, so this organ is also controlled by our circadian rhythm (Beesley et al. 2015).

Intense research is aimed at deciphering further mechanisms that act via these receptors and their effect on biological processes in the body (e.g., Yonei et al. 2010, Slominski et al. 2012, Wu et al. 2006). In addition, efforts are being made to identify additional melatonin production sites that might be responsible for the local effects of melatonin.

The melatonin receptors in the human body fulfill different functions depending on their location. For example, melatonin acts directly on our metabolism through its specific receptors in the gastrointestinal tract. In the brain, it controls cognitive performance and sleep behavior. In the cardiovascular system, it lowers heart rate and blood pressure (Söderquist et al. 2015).

Battle Substance in Cell Protection

One differentiates between receptor-dependent functions and those that are independent of a receptor. For example, the former include regulation of the circadian rhythm and thus support our sleep patterns, healthy bone growth, and protection against numerous diseases, including malignancies.

In addition to this receptor-dependent effect, melatonin also acts as a free radical scavenger independent of a receptor and protects the cells against damage resulting from oxidative stress (i.e., stroke or heart attack), UV rays, X-rays, or anemia (Reiter et al. 2014a). Also, the results of the receptor-independent effect of melatonin in animals apply equally in humans. (See Fig. 11.)

In addition to the pineal gland, other cells of our body have the ability to produce melatonin, especially in their mitochondria, the so-called power plants of the cell. The melatonin produced in this way is not released into the blood, as from the pineal organ, but acts directly on the spot. This often makes it impossible to prove how much melatonin is produced in these cells. Studies have shown that the mitochondria play an essential role in cell death (e.g., Juszczak and Drewa 2016, Letra-Vilela et al. 2016). Melatonin protects these cell organelles from attack by free radicals, which are responsible for the aging process and for numerous diseases, including diabetes, diseases of the brain and cardiovascular system, and cancer.

The protective qualities and positive effects of melatonin extend to all of our cells, regardless of whether the melatonin was formed on the spot, originated from the pineal gland, or was ingested as a supplement. For example, melatonin has the ability to reduce the toxic effects of chemotherapy, while also increasing the effectiveness of such treatment. Ongoing studies also provide the first promising results of melatonin in the fight against cancer. Melatonin, according to a study on its effect on prostate cancer, can positively influence or prevent the spread of tumor cells (Kiss and Ghosh 2016).

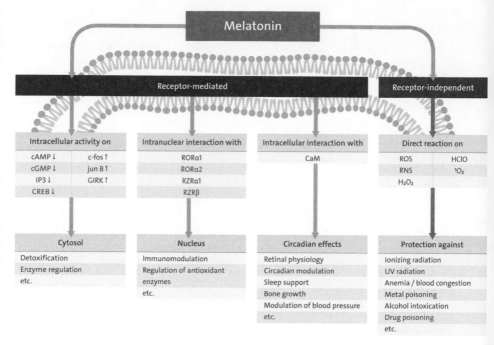

Fig. 11: Schematic representation of the intracellular effects of melatonin and its clinical effects (modified by Reiter et al. 2010b; Reiter et al. 2014a).

Free Radicals

For a long time, melatonin was known only as a hormone that required receptors for effector functions. It was then discovered that melatonin leads a double life and is also an extremely important and effective free radical scavenger. Melatonin has a high antioxidant effect and also intensifies the activity of the body's own antioxidative capacity (Reiter and Robinson 1995).

Free radicals damage our cells, cause diseases, and accelerate our aging process. As an antioxidant, melatonin acts against the destructive potential of free radicals and protects us from cataracts, stomach ulcers, Alzheimer's disease, Parkinson's disease, cancer, and AIDS, among others.

Free radicals are tiny fragments of molecules that cannot even be seen with an electron microscope. They are constantly formed in the body within nanoseconds and can disappear as quickly as they formed.

For example, the oxygen we inhale causes free radicals. Many metabolic processes in our bodies also produce free radicals. This natural process does not lead to dangerous consequences at first but serves to ward off infections, especially viruses and bacteria. In other words, free radicals arise where they are needed.

It becomes critical when one of these millions of casually formed oxygen molecules penetrating the body takes flight, and then another, and then another. Over time, these free radicals run amok, making trouble by killing individual cells, then whole cell structures, until finally their organ functions are affected.

Oxidative Stress

In addition to oxygen as the largest free radical generator, there are also external factors contributing to this damaging process. Radiation from UV light or radioactive sources, exhaust gases, smoking, alcohol, physical or psychological stress, and pollutants in our food—all of these contribute to the so-called oxidative stress. Our immune system is weakened, with the result that our body can no longer resist the invading germs.

To get a picture of the incredible number of free radicals, more than 10,000 free radicals are generated daily in every cell, primarily from endogenous sources in natural processes. If you are a smoker, the next example will not please you: every puff on the cigarette releases 100,000 free radicals in your body.

Increasingly, there are also indications for the involvement of oxidative stress in the development of heart disease, the development of arteriosclerosis (calcification of the arteries), and tissue damage after a stroke (Pandi-Perumal et al. 2013).

You may ask yourself now whether you—or your body—can actively contribute to combating free radicals. The good news is yes, you can. Vitamins and trace elements that you absorb through your diet help your body develop its antioxidative potential. Also, a healthy lifestyle with adequate sleep, and thus adequate melatonin, promotes the defense against free radicals.

During the day, we form more free radicals than at night. So if you are turning the night into the day or otherwise suppress your melatonin production, these damaging molecules also have more time to attack your cells. An imbalance will then occur, which can cause irreparable damage in your body.

Free Radicals and the Aging Process

When we are young and healthy, our bodies manage to keep the released molecules in check. As we age, however, it becomes increasingly difficult for our bodies to stop the oxidation. The antioxidant potential of your body decreases with increasing age, although the damaging attacks of free radicals remain the same or even increase.

Even if you are living in a lonely cabin in the mountains, away from exhaust fumes and pollution, the air you breathe and the sun that you are enjoying during the day will "supply" you with free radicals over time, resulting in damage to your body.

Free radicals may leave visible traces on the outside, from age spots on the body to sagging skin under the eyes or the formation of a double chin—but the most severe damage still occurs inside your body.

The brain, by the way, is most susceptible to free radicals. The damage they cause is irreparable and dramatic; just think about diseases like Alzheimer's, Parkinson's, or multiple sclerosis!

Melatonin Protects from Free Radicals

After all the not-so-nice remarks, finally some good news: every cell of your body can be protected by melatonin. It assists in the fight against free radicals especially during sleep, and particularly by protecting the cerebral nerve cells from oxidation.

It has been shown that melatonin is more potent in controlling free radicals than vitamin C and vitamin E (Reiter et al. 2014a)! The reason is that vitamin C does not reach the brain immediately, while melatonin penetrates very quickly and everywhere in every cell. The importance of this effect cannot be emphasized enough, as more than one hundred diseases of our time are associated with oxidative stress.

Numerous studies demonstrate the high antioxidant activity of melatonin in the fight against free radicals: in the treatment of cancer, cardiovascular diseases (e.g., myocardial infarction and stroke), metabolic diseases (e.g., Diabetes), inflammation, and apoptosis—programmed cell death, which is particularly important in chemotherapy. Furthermore, taken in a sufficient amount, melatonin is a very safe medication without any side effects (Reiter et al. 2016).

Melatonin: The Perfect Antioxidant

Within the total antioxidant potential of our body, melatonin is the most potent anti-free radical.

> It is effective globally, that is, in the whole body.
> It is very potent and substantially more effective than the vitamin C and E complex.
> It fights and neutralizes free radicals without becoming itself a radical.

> ❯ It protects the DNA from damage.
> ❯ It is completely nontoxic and can be used orally.

In its chemical structure, melatonin resembles a double ring. And it is precisely this ring structure that makes melatonin a unique hormone that acts as a perfect weapon against free radicals.

Ideally, the electrons of all atoms in our body occur in pairs. However, it can happen that they are on the road as a loner and looking for an electron partner. This constellation can be found in most free radicals, and they aggressively invade every atom or molecule in their vicinity in order to "steal" an electron, which means that the "robbed" atom or molecule no longer functions properly and thus can destroy the environment.

Melatonin can stop this process and eliminate the free radicals, for it is not only able to release electrons, but also to share them. It has a special gift that makes it such an effective antioxidant. Its ring structure neutralizes unpaired electrons; the ideal pair state of the electrons is restored, and free radicals no longer have a chance to wreak havoc.

Melatonin is the star among the so-called body-specific antioxidants, which can protect you against cataracts, stomach ulcers, and even cancer. Numerous studies have already been carried out with amazing results. Melatonin protects against free radicals, which are released during a stroke and can damage the brain much more than the stroke itself! In addition, it has been demonstrated that melatonin protects against radiation (e.g., X-rays). Melatonin also shows promising effects in cancer therapy (see, for example, Zamfir Chiru et al. 2014). A recent study summarized the great potential of melatonin as an antioxidant in its broad spectrum of activity. The study's authors' recommendation, in view of the excellent results achieved with melatonin, is that the further investigation of its mode of action(s) should be the focus of any biomedical research (Reiter et al. 2016).

Chronopharmacology: New Roads of Medicine

Have you ever taken the herbal supplement valerian in the morning? Try it, and you will be surprised by its stimulating and anxiety-reducing effect. In the evening, on the other hand, valerian displays its well-known calming and sleep-promoting effects.

The timing of the administration plays an essential role for all drugs; this is currently the subject of intensive research (e.g., Dallmann et al. 2016). Earlier studies show that a therapy that is correctly adapted to the time of the day can be much more effective or better tolerated than the conventional practice (i.e., one tablet morning, noon, and evening). This new field of research is called chronotherapy. For example, recent studies confirm that an individualized chronotherapy in the fight against cancer provides positive results for the future treatment of many forms of the disease (Innominato et al. 2014, Dulong et al. 2015).

Remember that cell division also follows a circadian rhythm. Researchers have now found that cancer drugs have an even greater effect when administered just at the moment the cells divide (Ortiz-Tudela et al. 2013). Another research group showed that the toxicity of chemotherapy could be reduced by a chronotherapeutically matched administration, and its efficacy could be simultaneously increased (Coudert et al. 2008).

Melatonin in Chronotherapy

Another study has investigated the consequences of anesthesia for the sleep of patients and found that narcotization during the day can adversely affect nocturnal melatonin production.

It is known that patients often suffer from sleep disorders after surgery. Chronopharmacology could have a supporting effect with melatonin for these patients (Ocmen et al. 2016).

An interesting result recently came from another study conducted by Spanish chronobiologists. For a long time, a link between hypertension and type 2 diabetes has been assumed. Both diseases are, so to speak, part of a common disease: the metabolic syndrome. Researchers have found that taking blood pressure medicines at a certain time can significantly reduce the risk of diabetes (Hermida et al. 2016). Whether melatonin can influence this therapeutic window is currently the subject of intensive research. However, what is certain is that melatonin can also reduce blood pressure and reduce the risk of diabetes.

What Is a Metabolic Syndrome?

The metabolic syndrome—also known as Syndrome X—identifies the following four risk factors that can lead to diseases such as type 2 diabetes, heart disease, and stroke:

> High blood sugar
> High cholesterol
> High blood pressure
> Large waist circumference

All in Good Time

It is not only in the case of valerian that the time at which the drug is taken determines its efficacy, but also when melatonin is taken for medication. It should also be noted whether the delivery method is fast or slow and how high the dosage is.

If you want to regulate your circadian rhythm by taking melatonin, you will be more likely to succeed by taking it regularly, in low dosage, and one or two hours before sleeping. In this case, it is a chronotherapy.

For example, if you want to use melatonin as an effective free radical scavenger following an acute medical incident such as a stroke, then you should be advised to take it immediately after the incident occurs and not wait for a certain time of day. Here, one speaks of a pharmacotherapy.

If you want to supplement melatonin because your body no longer produces it, you need a customized preparation that precisely adjusts your circadian rhythm. A chronobiologically correct hormone replacement therapy is then recommended to ensure that melatonin is available in sufficient quantities throughout the night phase.

Melatonin and the Main Fields of Application

From what has been shown to date, it is clear that melatonin can be an important tool to control many diseases, considering its impact on maintaining one's circadian rhythm. Even if not all the data available to date illustrate the full potential of this approach, one thing is already certain: there will be many changes in medicine in the foreseeable future. Before discussing the individual diseases in detail, we will provide a short overview.

Shift Work and Breast Cancer

As already mentioned, some circadian rhythm disorders are assumed to be contributing to some types of cancer—a reason why shift workers are much more likely to develop breast cancer (Sahar and Sassone-Corsi 2009). The World Health Organization (WHO) has therefore recently classified shift work as possibly cancer-promoting and postulated a direct relationship with disturbed melatonin production.

Researchers in Santa Cruz have discovered that a certain protein is likely responsible for the disordered rhythm in the tumor cells, which allows for the constant and unregulated growth of the malignant cells. Medications that are able to prevent that specific protein and restart the circadian rhythm are an important finding for the effective treatment of cancer. A complete and guaranteed cancer cure is not currently possible, but tumor growth can be significantly slowed (Michael et al. 2015). Therefore, melatonin can be used as an antitumor agent not only thanks to its cell-protective properties, but also because it is the most potent timer in our body.

Poisoning Due to Nephropathy

A recent study investigated multiple biological processes on which melatonin has an impact and concluded that melatonin can also be used to treat disorders such as obstructive nephropathy (when restricted blood flow causes kidney damage), which can cause severe poisoning of the body. Especially in clinical and surgical fields, the problem of free radicals being produced during injuries and obstruction of blood flow is widely acknowledged (Yildirim et al. 2016). Melatonin produces extremely positive effects by protecting the cell nucleus from free radicals. Since melatonin can penetrate into all cells, it could serve as a universal protection against such damage.

Social Jet Lag

If you took the test to determine your chronotype (see pp. 15–18), you know if you are more of a morning or evening person. If you fall into the "lark" category, you probably have no problems getting up in the morning and going to work early. The "owls" feel quite differently, because their individual daily rhythm often does not coincide with working hours. The circadian rhythm of the different types especially results in problems when working hours contradict their biorhythms, as is the case for morning people when they work the late shift.

A study recently investigated the individual sleep needs of typical chronotypes: the classic morning "larks" and the evening "owls." The evening types showed an even greater than previously assumed sleep deficit than the morning types. Their DLMO, or dim light melatonin onset (Lewy and Sack 1989), that is, the start of the nocturnal increase in melatonin, was markedly delayed, even on nonworkdays (Paine and Gander, 2016).

Scientists have coined a new name for this type of sleep deficit: "social jet lag," which is similar to the jet lag induced by traveling to different time zones. If the day and night rhythms during the week differ too much from those on the weekend, the body must permanently adapt itself to the new rhythm—with serious health consequences (cf., for example, Bonmati-Carrion et al. 2014, Wong et al. 2015, Matsumura et al. 2016). Again, these are the classical diseases of our time that increasingly occur, such as excess weight, diabetes, heart and cardiovascular disease, and cancer. A direct connection between the development of these diseases and disturbed melatonin rhythm can no longer be ignored.

Tips for Dealing With Social Jet Lag

First, even if a long night's sleep is the reward at the end of a long workweek for many—especially the night owls among you—it is best for your constant circadian rhythm if you also get up at your usual time on your days off.

Second, it is recommended not to turn the night into the day even on the weekend. It is important to keep your body in the same "time zone" all week for your sleep pattern and physical health (Rutters et al. 2014). Be aware that your body works like a clock. All processes happen every day, at the same time without interruption and without a difference, whether it is Tuesday, Friday, or Sunday. Try to make as few changes as possible to your body rhythm. You will feel better, and this will also have a positive impact on your long-term health.

Improving the Quality of Life

Studies have shown that melatonin improves the quality of life in old age and can prevent or mitigate diseases (e.g., Alzheimer's, arthritis, Parkinson's, and gastric ulcers) by interfering with the production of free radicals. It also provides protection against cancer cells, viruses, and bacteria that affect our aging process. Influenza viruses especially often have very serious and life-threatening consequences for the elderly. Melatonin strengthens your immune system and protects you against such infections.

Above all, melatonin supports restful sleep at night. It stabilizes the circadian rhythm, which leads to nocturnal resting and regeneration phases of all organs—a daily regeneration time for your body! There is something to the old adage "sleep well." For this, however, we need enough melatonin.

Protection for the Cardiovascular System

Older people with a melatonin deficiency often suffer from high blood pressure, which can lead to a stroke, diseases of the coronary arteries, and high cholesterol. Here, too, melatonin helps maintain healthy blood pressure by its antioxidant effect, not only against harmful cholesterol deposits, but also positively in regard to the cardiovascular system.

Heart attack and stroke are events of acute vessel occlusion. Melatonin has a great vasodilating ability and supports the circulation of blood with its regulating effect. It also protects the heart muscle, as well as the brain, from further damage as a perfect counteragent of free radicals. Recent studies also demonstrate its anti-inflammatory properties, which are particularly effective in the fight against atherosclerosis and associated hereditary diseases (Favero et al. 2014).

Mentally Fit in Old Age

Many people are afraid to lose their memory and cognitive abilities in old age. Medical research has established relationships among Alzheimer's, Parkinson's, and free radical damage. As we have seen, the older we get, the less resistance our bodies offer to ward off these tiny, malignant molecules. Melatonin intake can help protect the brain from this oxidative stress (Gutierrez-Cuesta et al. 2011). This is confirmed by numerous studies that have already successfully applied melatonin in the fight against brain-related diseases (e.g., Pandi-Perumal et al. 2013). As you already know, melatonin also helps to stabilize the circadian rhythm and thus the day-waking rhythm, which often gets out of sync in the elderly, thereby promoting memory performance (Chen et al. 2016a). One thing is known: a healthy sleep improves long-term memory and helps to solve complicated tasks better.

Digestion and Nutrition

Science suggests that melatonin also has a positive effect on body weight and energy turnover or metabolism. A study of women in menopause has shown that the intake of melatonin for the duration of one year had positive effects on their body composition. The women exhibited lower blood lipids and a higher lean body mass (i.e., higher "muscle mass"), which corresponds to the body weight minus the stored fat (Amstrup et al. 2016).

Melatonin also plays an important role in the synthesis, secretion, and effects of insulin. As a strong chronobiotic, melatonin is responsible for important metabolic processes. If the melatonin fluctuations are disturbed, this can lead not only to insomnia, but also to insulin resistance, glucose intolerance, and a marked circadian disorganization with further consequences, resulting in obesity and diabetes. This is the result of a study that also concluded that therapy with melatonin benefits the health of the whole body (Cipolla-Neto et al. 2014).

Numerous studies (for example, Giskeødegård et al. 2015; Davies et al. 2014) are constantly investigating the relationship between insufficient sleep and the occurrence of metabolic disorders, such as fatigue and diabetes. They all confirm that shortened sleep is a risk factor for a feeling of constant hunger, eating at night, and consuming too many calories. The consequence is a significant increase in weight, even to the point of morbid obesity. Sleep deprivation in men and women who were both normal and overweight contributed to a significant weight gain in all participants (Spaeth et al. 2015).

Diabetes

A disturbed circadian rhythm has long been associated with type 2 diabetes. Shift workers are especially at risk, in addition to many other serious illnesses. One study investigated this connection. For eight days, students followed a normal schedule of breakfast in the morning, dinner in the evening, and sleep at night. For the next four weeks, the schedule was the opposite. Breakfast was eaten in the evening, the participants worked during the night, ate dinner in the morning, and slept during the day. During this opposite period, their evening blood glucose levels were 17 percent higher than in the morning, despite the same breakfast on the plate (Morris et al. 2015). Why is that?

In the western diet, breakfast is usually very carbohydrate rich—think of your own habits and preferences for cereal or peanut butter and jelly sandwiches. While carbohydrates in the morning represent a workable task for our body and are often even useful (Fauteck and Platzer 2016), large quantities of them eaten in the evening lead to strong blood glucose fluctuations, which ultimately can lead to insulin resistance and thus diabetes.

Sleep and Nutrition

It is proven that a healthy sleep of seven to eight hours favors a healthy lifestyle and a healthy body weight. When did you last turn the night into the day and were not really awake in the morning? Do you remember the next day? Did you have cravings for sweets, chips, or other foods that are not necessarily known for their positive health benefits?

For some time now, researchers have been observing the relationship between sleep disorders and obesity. In people who sleep fewer than four hours, the body secretes the hunger-inducing hormone ghrelin and produces less leptin, a hunger-suppressing hormone. In short, sufficient sleep also leads to balanced eating habits and a healthy body. Evidence that melatonin has a positive effect on body weight and metabolism is increasing.

A recent study explored the differences between night owls and early risers and concluded that night owls tend to eat late in the day, smoke, exercise less, and develop diabetes or metabolic disorders such as the metabolic syndrome. Another very surprising result? Night owls also have to fear a negative impact on their health even when they get enough sleep and live a healthy lifestyle (Yu et al. 2015). So, what can typical night owls do to reduce these risk factors?

Tips for Night Owls

> Do not eat late in the evening or at night.
> Exercise regularly.
> Try to fall asleep early; melatonin helps you.
> An alarm clock with a light can help you wake up earlier in the morning.

The Vicious Cycle of Insulin

Studies with shift workers and the elderly have shown that sleep disturbances, melatonin deficiency, and metabolic disorders are related. However, recent studies also demonstrate that melatonin is able to modulate the synthesis and secretion of insulin, to protect the cells producing insulin from overload, thereby counteracting the development of type 2 diabetes (Peschke et al. 2015, Tuomi et al. 2016).

However, if melatonin is produced less—for example, due to the use of sleeping pills, beta-blockers, alcohol, nocturnal light, or increasing age—this leads to long-term insulin resistance and type 2 diabetes. The reason is that melatonin acts on specific receptors on the pancreas, which is responsible for the release of insulin, thus preventing insulin from being released at night. However, if too little melatonin is produced for the reasons mentioned, a vicious cycle is set in motion. Through the release of insulin even at night, the blood glucose level drops, and we get hungry. The nightly walk to the refrigerator is then preprogrammed. A further consequence of melatonin deficiency is that the body accustoms itself to the permanently increased insulin and is resistant, even during the day, which often leads to diabetes with all its accompanying symptoms.

Nocturnal food intake in itself also has indirect negative effects on our sleep and insulin production, similar to stress. If you want to do something good for your health and slow down your aging process, avoid heavy foods and carbohydrates that stimulate insulin in the evening. And above all, leave the refrigerator closed at night. These measures support your brain functions at the same time. A study has confirmed that diet—both what you eat as well as the timing of your meals—affects the performance of your brain (Leheste and Torres 2015). Less is thus often more.

Depression

Studies have shown that light therapy can help with depression—and even shows a greater effect than some drugs. Since the 1970s, this relationship has been known mainly for seasonal depressions. Recent studies confirm the positive effect of light therapy, even for severe depressions that are not dependent on the seasons. A study with 122 depressed patients showed astounding effects when patients were exposed to bright light for only half an hour a day (Lam et al. 2016)—a result that provides hope for many people that is cost-effective and without side effects. This therapy primarily influences the circadian rhythm and thus melatonin production.

Melatonin for Depression

Many studies have also confirmed melatonin can have a positive effect on many symptoms during the treatment of depression. Particularly good results have been obtained in the treatment of sleep disorders (Li et al. 2013). Positive effects after melatonin administration were also observed in patients suffering from winter depression. Their mood improved markedly as the melatonin synchronized the biological rhythm to the changed light conditions during the winter months or to those rhythms of people who did not suffer from this disease.

And recently, an investigation has shown that depression can be predicted by the melatonin levels contained in saliva (Sundberg et al. 2016). You can see the very strong correlation among depression, melatonin, and altered sleep.

Light Stimulates the Internal Clock

Light therapy also shows a healing effect for patients not suffering from depression. Even in the case of shift workers or people who suffer from jet lag, the solution to their day-night rhythm problem can lie in the correct light supply. Special light boxes or devices can help bring the inner clock back into the right cycle and adapt to the new environmental conditions.

For some time, light therapy has been successfully used in circadian-rhythm-adjustment disorders, such as in shift work or jet lag. It also has positive effects in mood swings. One study has recently revealed that intermittent light, which temporarily turns off and on, is particularly effective at bringing the circadian rhythm back on the right course (Najjar and Zeitzer 2016).

Studies with school children showed that the right light source can also increase concentration and performance. For this purpose, a new, brighter lighting was installed in a school class, which more closely matched natural sunlight and contained more blue light. The results were astonishing: all students achieved better results in tests, and their learning abilities were greater than those of the comparative class with conventional blue-deficient room lighting. The children also reported they had slept better during the night and had awakened in the morning feeling fresher and more rested (Keis et al. 2014).

Healing Light for the Elderly

The influence of light on elderly people was examined by another study (Karami et al. 2016). The inhabitants of a nursing home were exposed to daylight in the morning from 9 to 10 a.m. and late in the afternoon from 4 to 5 p.m. The results were remarkable: all subjects showed regulated day-night rhythms after daily sunbathing.

The scientists concluded that if elderly people are exposed to daylight every day, sleep phases can be lengthened and circadian rhythms corrected. Other positive effects are that anxiety and insomnia are significantly reduced (Karami et al. 2016).

Light Therapy Also for Visually Impaired People?

You may now wonder whether light therapy can also have an effect on the visually impaired. What is certain is that these people are most affected by chronodisruption, much more than people with normal vision, or even some falsely diagnosed, completely blind people!

Special photoreceptors in the eyes are particularly sensitive and react to every slight change in light. It is precisely with this group of persons that a light therapy with individually matched devices shows excellent effects. However, this only works if their photoreceptors, which we call "nonvisual vision," are still present. In the case of many visually impaired people, although they can still recognize something, these receptors are no longer present, which means that they no longer perceive light. In this case, the pineal gland, and thus the entire rhythm, is no longer adjusted to the day-night rhythm. In the case of supposedly completely blind people in whom these receptors still function, though they otherwise consciously no longer see anything, light can still function as a timer, and there is no chronodisruption.

Electromagnetic Fields

The fact that electromagnetic fields are extremely harmful to humans is something you may have already experienced when talking on the phone for too long; your head feels heated and booming, but this is not due to the fact that your mobile phone is too close to your ear.

Studies have shown that electromagnetic fields can cause cancer, lead to miscarriages, trigger depression, and so forth. It is also assumed that a constant exposure lowers melatonin levels. Numerous studies are in progress, all of which are investigating the effect—even if it's weak—of electromagnetic fields on melatonin production (e.g., Seifpanahi-Shabani et al. 2016).

Recently, a study investigated the effects of electro-smog on rats and their circadian rhythm. It was found that environmental stress factors significantly interfere with the release of melatonin (Yuan et al. 2016). The exact nature of this relationship, however, is still the subject of intensive research.

Electromagnetism in the Household

How many electromagnetic fields are there in your household? Think of your microwave, stove, TV, computer and monitor, baby monitor, and so forth. In each household, these and other devices are an integral part of the surroundings. So how can you protect yourself from them? And is this protection at all possible or necessary?

What you should know: the farther away you are from power lines, the better, because of the lower the risk for you. When your dishwasher is operating, leave the room. If you are still in the kitchen, even if you are only a few feet away, the electromagnetic field strength is measurable.

But what about the alarm clock next to the bed? Or the mobile phone on the night table? Experts advise keeping a distance of at least one arm's length. It is important and would be ideal, however, that your bedroom be completely free from electromagnetic fields. Then your sleep will be relaxing and healthy, and the melatonin production in your body will be completely undisturbed.

Disturbances of Healthy Melatonin Production

As you probably already suspect, there are a number of factors that can interfere with our melatonin production. At the top of the list is artificial light, which we can barely avoid today. Even the smallest amount, especially of blue light, is sufficient to block the activity of the pineal gland. Light can not only suppress production, but it can also shift the time at which the pineal gland is active, which results in the release of reduced melatonin at the wrong time.

In addition, there are many other factors that affect the function of the pineal gland.

Drugs

Beta-blockers, which are used as blood pressure agents, are among the handful of drugs that affect melatonin formation. As their name suggests, they block the beta-receptor, which is important in starting melatonin production.

Additional drugs that affect sleep are benzodiazepines, or antidepressants. They stimulate sleep but suppress the body's melatonin release. In other words, by taking a sleeping pill, you block the production of your own sleep regulator.

If you have to take certain antidepressants on a regular basis, your melatonin level may be drastically reduced, or the time of melatonin release may be postponed.

Studies with aspirin have shown that it can also partly suppress melatonin release (Murphy et al. 1994). Many patients in the studies report problems during and after sleep. Long-term use, especially in the evening, prevents melatonin from protecting you from numerous diseases by acting as a free radical scavenger.

Paracetamol, when administered in the evening, has been shown to inhibit melatonin formation to the same extent as ibuprofen and aspirin. If, on the other hand, these products are taken early during the day, they have almost no effect on the production of nocturnal melatonin. One way to prevent these drugs from affecting your sleep is to ask your doctor if you can take these either in the morning or during the day, and at the latest before dinner. If aspirin is to be taken in the evening for health reasons, it is advisable to consider whether the benefits of aspirin are greater than its melatonin-inhibitory effect and whether this inhibition cannot be corrected by external melatonin.

Related Products

Do you like to have a cup of coffee in the evening, or do you refrain from doing so because you would have trouble falling asleep? Coffee has long been known to have a negative impact on sleep. If you intake caffeine, you have probably already observed this in yourself. If you know people who do not mind drinking coffee in the evening, do not be fooled! Many studies have shown that most people sleep considerably worse after coffee consumption, even if they are not aware of this. An investigation has shown that a cup of coffee that is drunk at 8 p.m. can delay the melatonin production by several hours. Only a few people are able to break down coffee so quickly that no negative effect is produced.

This also applies to black tea, caffeinated lemonades, and, unfortunately, certain chocolates. Some chocolates can contain up to 30 mg of caffeine at 40 g of chocolate, but others contain significantly less caffeine. Very dark chocolates, which are considered healthy when enjoyed in moderation, contain a very high proportion of tryptophan, which in turn can have a mood-improving effect. In those who are no longer producing melatonin from tryptophan—for example, in the elderly—this consumption can lead to sleep disturbances.

All the health-damaging effects of nicotine need not be mentioned here. Smoking lowers the melatonin level, as does alcohol, which may help in the short term to help you fall asleep but can disturb your circadian rhythm in the long run (Prosser and Glass 2015).

B Vitamins Support Melatonin Production

In addition to a healthy circadian rhythm, vitamins and minerals, like vitamins B3, B12, and B6, are also important for our melatonin production. These are contained in bananas, carrots, crabs, salmon, liver, lentils, rice, soybeans, sunflower seeds, tuna, wheatgrass, wheat bran, and wheat flour. Doctors recommend taking vitamin B6 earlier in the day, because it has a stimulating effect right after consumption. The remaining B vitamins should be taken in the evening. Calcium and magnesium are also very important for melatonin production. Similarly, tryptophan supports melatonin distribution and is contained in cottage cheese, chicken liver, pumpkin seeds, breakfast cereals with milk, turkey meat, chicken, tofu, almonds, peanuts, brewer's yeast, milk, ice cream, and yogurt. Unfortunately, a lack of melatonin caused by too little tryptophan can only be compensated by diet at a young age. In the elderly, tryptophan taken up through food can no longer be converted into melatonin during the night and is therefore more likely to have stimulating effects.

Plants Also Contain Melatonin

Did you know that melatonin is not exclusively found in humans? It also exists in plants and is contained in measurable concentrations in oats, sweet corn, rice, ginger, tomatoes, bananas, and barley. Especially if eaten before bedtime, these foods support melatonin production and, thus, sleep. However, you cannot cover the daily requirement of melatonin with just your diet, because, for example, you would have to eat 200 kg of tomatoes to make your melatonin level rise measurably!

Tips for a Melatonin-Friendly Lifestyle

> Spend more time in sunlight or very bright artificial light.
> Sleep long enough that you are rested in the morning.
> Avoid bright lights at night.
> Do not expose yourself to electromagnetic fields.
> Do not smoke or drink alcohol.
> Do not take any medication that affects melatonin levels.
> Take breaks often.
> Avoid frequent air travel over many time zones.
> Avoid shift work.

II. MELATONIN IN PRACTICE

Melatonin, the Multitalent

A healthy circadian rhythm and a healthy melatonin level, in particular, have many positive effects on your health. Over the last twenty years, numerous clinical trials have tested the therapeutic benefits of melatonin in various medical fields and have shown how effective this hormone can be in combating various diseases (Sánchez-Barceló et al. 2010).

Wide Spectrum of Effects

The positive effects of melatonin have been proven many times, not only for healthy sleep and a controlled day-night rhythm, but also for epilepsy, jetlag, diabetes (especially type 2), neuropsychiatric disorders (e.g., Alzheimer's and Parkinson's), and even in acute events (e.g., stroke and heart attack). Melatonin relieves stress, pain, and metabolic disturbances, and it increases blood circulation, which has already achieved good success, particularly in the elderly. In cancer treatment, it promotes the efficacy of chemo- and radiation therapy, while simultaneously reducing their negative side effects (Emet et al. 2016). As you can see, melatonin is indeed a molecule with diverse properties, which is why it is sometimes referred to as the "Swiss army knife" in scientific circles.

Research groups all over the world are working hard to investigate which other serious diseases can be associated with circadian rhythmic disorders in order to discover new areas of application for melatonin. What is already established is that melatonin not only achieves good results as a monotherapy, but also shows positive effects when coupled with conventional treatments (Rivara et al. 2015).

Circadian Disorders and Their Clinical Significance

Disorders of the normal circadian rhythm are almost always associated with a disturbed melatonin signal, whether it is because at night too little melatonin is released or it's released at the wrong time. Irrespective of the cause of these disorders, clear connections with certain diseases can be identified.

Hormones of Melatonin

A lack of melatonin affects those hormones whose daily rhythmic release is also synchronized by the melatonin signal. For example, if age-dependent melatonin production decreases too early in women, it can trigger a very early onset of menopause. A lower melatonin level means that the sex hormones are no longer sufficiently produced and, above all, no longer released rhythmically.

This also applies to the production of the growth hormone HGH—human growth hormone—also called the "vitality hormone." It makes us feel good, protects our bones and immune system, and plays an important role in burning fat. If melatonin is absent, the increased evening production of HGH is reduced or massively disturbed.

Inadequate melatonin also affects the liver and the work that is usually done at night. The result is insulin resistance, which can lead to diabetes. In addition, the urge to urinate at night remains as strong as during the day. Because of the lack of melatonin, a special hormone that inhibits urine production (antidiuretic hormone, ADH) is missing.

Melatonin deficiency has a special effect on our brains, negatively affecting our nightly repair mechanisms. For example, the storage of information to our long-term memory, which takes place predominantly at night, is no longer supported. A serious consequence is that we become more susceptible to early onset dementia (Alagiakrishnan 2016). As you can see, a low nocturnal melatonin signal begins a cycle that affects our entire body system.

Melatonin in Circadian Rhythm Disorders

When the circadian rhythm is disturbed, melatonin is often released at the wrong time, regardless of whether it is sufficient or not. This is the case among young people who want to stay up late but do not want to get up in the morning. In this group, the melatonin begins its release very late in the evening but remains at a very high level until the early morning hours.

An extended or delayed melatonin signal was also detected during winter depression or the delayed sleep onset syndrome. We will return to both of these diseases later on. Another rhythm disorder is present in the non-24 syndrome, i.e., a sleep-wake disorder that occurs especially in blind people, in shift work, and in jet lag.

The modern, chronotherapeutic approach has proven itself effective in these rhythm disorders by way of melatonin (usually taken in the evening), drugs containing melatonin agonists (which works especially well for blind people), and morning light therapy.

What Are Agonists and Antagonists?

The so-called melatonin agonists are active substances that attach themselves to specific melatonin receptors and activate them. They are chemically related to melatonin but do not occur in nature. Three active ingredients currently used are agomelatine, ramelteon, and tasimelteon.

Antagonists, on the other hand, block the melatonin receptors. There is currently only one antagonist—Luzindole—that is only used in the laboratory.

Melatonin in Age-Related Deficits

A deficit of melatonin can have several causes as a person ages. We have already seen how harmful blue light is for melatonin production and for our sleep. Likewise, some medicines strongly influence or inhibit our melatonin metabolism, including beta-blockers, aspirin, and ibuprofen. Caffeine and alcohol abuse also interfere with the nocturnal release of melatonin.

In addition to these factors, there are diseases that negatively affect our melatonin budget, including the metabolic syndrome, which seems to block the rhythmic release of melatonin.

In depression, a serotonin deficiency is responsible for the lack of melatonin. Recall that melatonin is formed from the happiness hormone serotonin, which in turn is produced by tryptophan. Imbalances within the trio have an effect on each individual player.

We should not forget that stress also has an adverse effect on our melatonin level. The increased adrenaline that our body distributes in stressful situations blocks the pineal gland, which in turn is responsible for melatonin production.

In all these cases of a deficit, a classic hormone replacement therapy is recommended; melatonin must be physically substituted to restore the circadian rhythm.

Melatonin as a Drug

Melatonin doses of over 1 mg can only be obtained with a prescription in German-speaking countries (Germany, Austria, and Switzerland), as well as in some other EU countries. This is different in the United States, where melatonin is freely available in all doses and can be found on the shelves of almost every pharmacy.

Dosages and Possible Side Effects

To date, there are still no uniform guidelines for melatonin dosages for specific diseases. In the most diverse clinical trials published so far, researchers have used dosages of 0.5 mg or less, or up to 25 mg or more—a very wide range that makes it difficult to compare the results.

In addition, these different dosages were all administered in various forms of tablets or capsules (e.g., fast-release, slow-release, chronobiologically combined/pulsatile), so that comparability is also not unequivocal. One study investigated whether an oral or intravenous administration of melatonin resulted in different serum levels. The result: there are no significant clinical differences, with the exception that in the intravenous administration, more melatonin was found in the blood than after oral administration (Andersen et al. 2016). If melatonin is used as a tablet or capsule, about 30 to 40 percent of the melatonin is absorbed. After about twenty-five minutes, half of the melatonin taken as a pill is already broken down, so there is no longer any significant melatonin after approximately 2.5 hours. These characteristics must be considered, for example, if melatonin is to be administered to the elderly for six to seven hours from the outside, i.e., as a tablet or capsule. Dosage regimens must be chosen if melatonin is to be delivered continuously over a prolonged period.

To summarize all the results so far available (see, for example, Harpsøe et al. 2015), consider the following dosage recommendations:

Chronotherapeutic Approach: Melatonin as a Timer

In the case of chronotherapy, where patients want to adjust their internal clock, melatonin amounts of 0.5 mg to 1 mg are sufficient as fast-release dosage forms.

Also, a pulsatile (pulse-like administration of up to 3 mg) administration was shown as effective. This applies to those who suffer from shift work and jet lag in particular. The administration time depends on the new time zone in the case of jet lag or the corresponding rest phase during shift work.

Hormonetherapeutic Approach: Deficit Is Balanced

This is a classical substitution therapy useful in the elderly. A pulsatile administration form is usually best, a delayed-release is less effective, and a fast-release dosage form is least effective. Doctors and nurses should ensure that melatonin be given to the patient in sufficient quantities for about six to seven hours during the night. This is achieved by an amount of 3 mg, which can also be increased to 6 mg without any problem. The ideal time to take it is around 30 minutes before bedtime but always before midnight, so as not to cause any rhythm shifts.

Pharmacological Therapy Approach: Melatonin for Acute Emergency

In the case of supporting therapies, such as those for a stroke or myocardial infarction, higher dosages are required. In the earlier studies, quantities of up to 50 mg and more were used successfully as an immediate measure, and specifically as a fast-release form of melatonin. The administration took place immediately after the occurrence of the event, independent of the time of day.

It is also advisable to use higher doses for concurrent therapy in tumor patients. Whether these are to be administered in the evening is still controversial but very likely. In the case of radiation therapy, doses of 15 mg need to be administered shortly before the treatment.

Other indications, such as epilepsy, neuroprotection, and rhythm stabilization, are most likely to benefit from a pulsatile or delayed dosage form of 3–6 mg in the evening. It should be noted that children are more likely to need a higher dose than adults.

Melatonin without Side Effects

Although not many studies on possible side effects are available, all studies show that melatonin is very well tolerated. A meta-analysis of several studies, which administered predominantly 10 mg and more, showed that the frequency and severity of reported adverse reactions were identical to those seen in patients who received a placebo (Seabra et al. 2000). (See Fig. 12.)

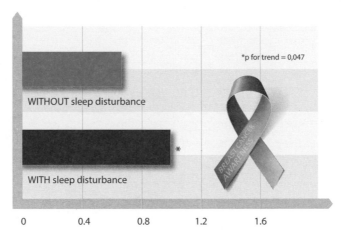

Fig. 12: Relative breast cancer risk in postmenopausal women in relation to their sleeping habits (modified according to Wu et al. 2008).

All previous studies lead to the conclusion that side effects may occur only if melatonin is taken incorrectly. This means that when melatonin is taken at the wrong time, one can become drowsy, leading to a decrease in concentration and possibly affecting visual acuity—symptoms that may occur with any sleep deficit. Intensive dreaming was also reported.

In very rare cases, a paradoxical effect of extreme insomnia occurs in patients. This is most likely due to contamination of the drug during preparation, which can cause allergies, but it has not yet been demonstrated. Intolerance of melatonin itself could also be the cause.

Extremely high doses administered in animal experiments show the following:

- Melatonin is absolutely nontoxic.
- Melatonin is by no means carcinogenic, but rather has a positive effect in the fight against cancer.
- Melatonin has no negative effect on the fetus.

Today, melatonin that is sold is synthetic. It corresponds 100 percent to the body's melatonin and is not genetically modified.

When Is Additional Melatonin Needed?

> If you suffer from a circadian rhythmic disorder, such as jet lag or shift work
> If you have a melatonin deficiency for various reasons
> If you want to achieve a pharmacological effect, such as alleviating stroke symptoms or assisting with radiation therapy in cancer treatment

Up to 1 mg melatonin is freely available in many European countries. Products with more than 1 mg require a prescription almost everywhere in Europe.

Measuring Melatonin

You have heard it several times: melatonin is released into the blood from the pineal gland at night and distributed to all tissues. As soon as it is broken down in the body, the byproducts are excreted primarily in one's urine. Because of this circulation, melatonin can be chemically detected in all body fluids, such as the blood, saliva, and cerebrospinal fluid. Measuring the amounts of byproducts in urine can serve to determine whether melatonin is produced in sufficient quantity and at the right time. However, not all body fluids are equally suitable for these analyses.

Blood measurements have proven to be the most suitable, since the daily changes of melatonin are most clearly reflected in them and it is there where the highest concentrations are reached. However, in order to create a complete day profile, or at least a complete profile during the night, blood collection is required every hour. This is a very complex procedure, as the blood sampling should be done in almost complete darkness. In practice, these examinations are carried out mainly in specialist hospitals, where blood is drawn regularly from the vein via a continuous catheter; and the people who carry out these withdrawals use special equipment, such as night vision goggles. This is the only way to ensure that the patient not be exposed to any light that would adversely affect the production of melatonin and thus affect the result of the measurement.

The so-called DLMO (dim light melatonin onset)—the time at dusk when the pineal gland starts to release melatonin—is a special measurement that can be determined by taking blood samples. It is precisely this value that provides information on whether the personal daytime rhythm is shifted forward or backward, as in the case of jet lag or during shift work. If it is known whether a change is present, this rhythm can be adjusted again by adequate melatonin or light therapy.

Partial or complete deficits of melatonin release can also be detected by these measurements, or else by determining the melatonin content in the saliva. For this purpose, the patient delivers several saliva samples that are distributed over the day or night. The advantage of this method is that this sample can be collected on an outpatient basis (e.g., at home). However, the patients should not be exposed to excessive light during the night, but rather stay in rooms with slightly darkened night lights or lamps with red light. One disadvantage of this method is that because the melatonin is passing from the blood into the saliva, the concentration in saliva is only ⅓ of what is found within the blood; therefore the melatonin concentration is determined to be very low. The patient should not consume any food or liquids about 30 minutes before the sample is taken, to avoid contamination. It is very difficult to determine DLMO or rhythm shifts using this method, because it can be very difficult to define, if at all.

The third method, detection by urinalysis, is only suitable to determine whether melatonin is produced at night at all. This method cannot clearly demonstrate when and how much melatonin is released over time. One collects all the urine from 8 a.m. to 8 p.m. and compares this sample with the one collected between 8 p.m. and 8 a.m.

For all measuring methods, it must be noted that no uniform standard values have yet been defined. This is due to the changing melatonin production over the course of our lives.

In many cases, a partial or complete melatonin deficiency can already be determined by an accurate patient survey. For example, if sleep disturbances or premature awakenings are reported, the presumption is that the release of melatonin starts too late or ceases too early. If these people are treated with a correct melatonin therapy and if the symptoms disappear within a few days, the initial suspicion of a melatonin deficiency is confirmed (Almeida et al. 2011).

Melatonin in Various Pathologies

Even if the effect of melatonin is still the subject of ongoing research, many studies already show the positive effects of this hormone on our bodies and the treatment of many diseases.

Sleep

Our sleep fulfills many functions. It is outstandingly significant for our brain and many important processes in our body, such as our memory capacity. Sleep helps our organs to regenerate at night and is essential for our metabolism (Kunz 2006).

What is most important is high-quality sleep. You certainly know days when you wake up refreshed early in the morning, full of energy for the tasks you have to do. Each of us, however, also experiences days when getting up is difficult. You just can't get going, your concentration leaves something to be desired—as well as your mood. Often, the metabolism also seems to have come out of balance, and digestion does not work properly.

A somewhat older study investigated the impact of sleep deprivation on young, healthy adults. For this, male subjects slept only four hours per night over six days. As a result, they developed symptoms and risk factors for diabetes, obesity, and cardiovascular diseases (Spiegel et al. 1999).

Sleep Affects Our Immune System

Sleep also affects our immune system and strengthens our so-called immune memory, as confirmed by a recent study (Westermann et al. 2015). If bacteria or viruses that have previously penetrated our body try to attack again, the T cells activate and stimulate the immune system to destroy the intruder before it can cause a disease. Researchers have now found that people who sleep too little are four times more likely to get the flu, colds, and so forth, because their immune system is weakened by sleep deficit (Prather et al. 2015).

"It is no small art to sleep: For that purpose you must keep awake all day," wrote Friedrich Nietzsche in *Thus Spoke Zarathustra* (1883–85). Anyone who has ever had to struggle with falling asleep or who knows sleep disorders too well will agree with these wise words. To get enough sleep is important in order to feel well rested and lead a healthy life. And that is completely independent of how old you are.

It is important that you become aware of what is going on in your body during sleep and what influence it has on your physical and mental health.

What Happens during Sleep? The First Sleep Cycle

Sleep occurs in cycles. In the first sleep phase, the clarity of consciousness is increasingly restricted. Many people experience optical, dreamlike impressions in this murky transitional state between waking and sleeping. At the same time, the eyeballs begin to move very slowly back and forth. Some people also show fine twitches of the eyelids when they fall asleep. There may also be violent convulsions of individual limbs or of the entire body.

You probably know this feeling when you suddenly wake up, because your hand or foot has moved uncontrolled. These are perfectly normal signs, probably due to a change in the motor control system during sleep.

The beginning of the second sleep stage is considered as the actual time sleep begins. The duration of time between bedtime and the start of sleep (or sleep latitude) is about 10–15 minutes in healthy adults. Normally, the sleep deepens gradually from this point onward and goes into deep sleep, then further still into the first REM sleep, which concludes the first sleep cycle of the night. (See Fig. 13.)

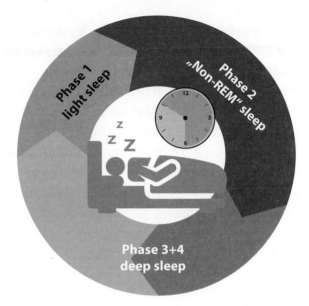

Fig. 13: Schematic representation of the different sleep phases.

The Other Sleep Cycles and the REM Phases

During one night, the individual sleep stages are repeated several times. The maximum duration of deep sleep occurs during the first sleep cycle. During the course of one night, you sleep through four to five such cycles, each lasting about one and a half hours. The REM episodes increase continuously during the night from about 5 to 10 minutes to 20 to 30 minutes. The eye movement density also increases noticeably in REM sleep. The intensification of REM sleep is accompanied by an intensification of many other physiological processes, such as dreaming. In REM sleep, one is often active and emotionally dreaming, whereas in the remaining sleep phases, dreaming does not occur.

REM sleep is also referred to as paradoxical sleep. Interestingly, the EEG of people in REM sleep hardly differs from those in the waking state. Furthermore, we are most likely to remember the content of the dreams when we wake up during the REM phase.

The Functions of the Individual Sleep Phases

Light sleep

> Pulse, respiratory rate, and blood pressure drop
> Slow eye movements (Phase 1)
> Transition to deep sleep
> Makes about 50 percent of total sleep

Deep sleep

> Very low frequencies in the EEG
> Very important for regeneration
> Reduced brain activity
> Very hard to wake up
> Brain "cleans up," i.e., processes the information received during the day
> Makes about 25 percent of total sleep
> Mostly within the first half of the night

REM sleep

> Increase of pulse, respiratory rate, and blood pressure
> Lots of brain activity (sensations, emotions, visual cortex)
> Areas that check for plausibility and reality are not active
> Spatial awareness and movement control deactivated
> Drive control, information processing, stress management
> Largely in the second half of the night

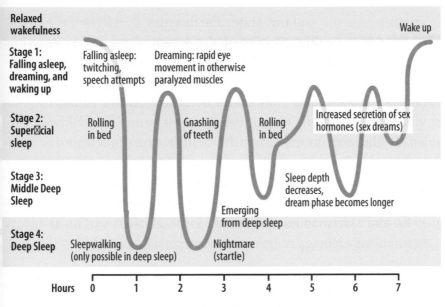

Fig. 14: Cycles of different sleep stages.

Sleep as Brain Doping

You recognize the many important effect of sleep on the processes in our body, on our health, and on our daily condition. Therefore, we are well advised to get adequate and healthy sleep. However, what we often forget is that sleep is also a very effective form of brain doping. Our brain needs these rest times urgently to regenerate, to process and store all the information that is recorded during a day, and to support our memory performance every new day.

Many people over the age of sixty and even younger people have difficulties with their memory ability. There is also a large number of studies linking sleep and memory consolidation—a very complex process of storing and retrieving information (Trinder et al. 2001, Rasch and Born 2013).

How are you on days when you have a short night behind you or woke up several times without being able to fall asleep again? Do you find it hard to concentrate? Are you having trouble retrieving what you learned the day before? No wonder—your brain did not have the time and peace to gather, organize, and store important information in the long-term memory department.

It has been shown that in the case of disturbed sleep, demonstrably fewer memories are retained, and even memories from the previous day are deleted! So be aware that you can use your sleep for optimal learning because learning is transferred to long-term memory during healthy sleep. For example, vocabulary and formulas are strengthened in the first half of the night, while motor skills are improved in the second half. Often, after awakening, we can recognize new relationships and gain solutions and insights. Do you want to promote your creativity? Then make sure you get a restful night's sleep!

Sleep Disorders

We've already seen that different people need different amounts of sleep. Nevertheless, a healthy and ideal sleep time is about seven to eight hours. Infants and children need more sleep. Even many adults are best off when they sleep nine hours.

Sleep disorder refers to a state when a person gets fewer than six hours sleep per night over a period of at least six months. The consequences can be fatal, because chronic sleep disturbances in an average of three out of seven nights considerably increases the likelihood of myocardial infarction, stroke, diabetes, vascular diseases, and obesity.

About 35 percent of the total population suffers from sleep disorders. This is made more difficult by the fact that only about 30 percent of those affected are seeking a doctor's help to deal with this health-endangering situation (see test 2).

Tips for Your Perfect Sleep Hygiene
> Sleep seven hours to stay healthy, not gain weight, and become more intelligent.
> Go to sleep at the same time every night.
> Wake up at the same time every morning.
> Do not engage in excessive physical activity before going to bed.
> Eat at least three hours before going to bed and avoid heavy foods.
> Let the evening end with quiet activities.
> Avoid sleeping aids.
> Avoid alcohol.
> Do not expose yourself to blue light (e.g., mobile phones, tablets, or TV).

The Right Sleep Duration

Minimal disturbances while falling asleep or during sleep, and even too much sleep, can affect the quality of our sleep. The results of a study at the University of Pennsylvania, consisting of a huge data volume of more than 130,000 people with an average age of 46 years, was analyzed for the first time. The conclusion of the research team? Even in the case of slight disturbances of sleep, the risk of being overweight increased by 35 percent, of diabetes by 54 percent, and of cardiovascular diseases by 98 percent. The risk of a stroke doubled (Irwin et al. 2016).

Test 2: This Is How You Recognize That You Have a Sleep Disorder

❭ You have problems falling asleep.
○ Not at all ○ Rarely ○ Frequently ○ Very frequently

❭ You wake up several times during the night.
○ Not at all ○ Rarely ○ Frequently ○ Very frequently

❭ You have problems getting into gear in the morning.
○ Not at all ○ Rarely ○ Frequently ○ Very frequently

❭ You have a strong need for sleep during the day.
○ Not at all ○ Rarely ○ Frequently ○ Very frequently

❭ You are often irritated and tense.
○ Not at all ○ Rarely ○ Frequently ○ Very frequently

Evaluation: If you have marked frequently/very frequently more than three times, you most likely have a sleep disorder. Please consult your doctor.

Catching Up on Sleep?

You know the situation: on the previous day, you went to bed late, and you want to make up for your sleep deficit with a nap the next day so you are fit for the rest of the day. This is an unfortunate misconception, because nocturnal sleep cannot be caught up! Sleep during the night has a completely different sleep structure than that during the day. For example, our body temperature does not drop during the day as it does at night, so it does not help to try to ameliorate a long-term sleep deficit with naps during the day. This does not mean that a midday sleep cannot be useful, either.

Naps, Siestas, and So Forth

Are you tired after lunch or in the afternoons and want to have a short nap? Then you are like a lot of people who feel refreshed, powerful, and fit after a shorter sleep phase in the day.

In our culture, naps are more associated with children. Southern countries with a hot climate know the *siesta* as a fixed component during the day that promotes health and productivity. Also, in Japan, *inemuri*—a short nap during meetings, sometimes just on the street corner or in the subway—is an important cultural component. In some Asian countries, there is even a legal claim on the midday sleep.

How healthy is a short nap during the day? In science, the opinions are divided. There are short "naps," "power napping," or a sleep phase of up to 45 minutes at certain times of the day. They do not influence the circadian rhythm, since they have a completely different sleep structure. They are even health promoting, as a recent study has found (Kallistratos 2015). People who take naps tend to have lower blood pressure and need fewer medications for hypertension. In addition, these people often have better memory and are more attentive after lunch, increasing their productivity and making them less vulnerable to accidents.

Nonetheless, it is not recommended to take a nap every day. Some feel even tired after the short sleep and do not even get into gear at all. Others sleep too long and have difficulties with falling asleep in the evening.

Napping like a Pro

> Do not sleep for more than 10–30 minutes.
> Plan your nap: When are you tired?
> Look for a quiet, comfortable place.
> Give yourself a few minutes to wake up.

Study: Melatonin Promotes Deep Sleep

Sleep disturbances are currently mainly treated with benzodiazepines such as temazepam and their derivatives, such as zolpidem. A study investigated the effect these drugs actually have on sleep and compared these to the effect of melatonin. Healthy women and men between the ages of 55 and 64 participated in the study. They were given slowly releasing melatonin, temazepam, and zolpidem on different nights, and researchers subsequently compared the influence of these preparations on deep sleep.

The results showed that slowly releasing melatonin did not adversely affect the normal deep-sleep phase in these subjects. Only a small, but rather positive, influence could be observed in just the first third of the night. On the other hand, temazepam and zolpidem significantly reduced deep sleep during the night (Arbon et al. 2015). In addition, it is known that many benzodiazepines suppress the body's production of melatonin and can even cause sleep disturbances.

The Effects Too Little Sleep Can Have on You:

> You feel powerless and have to struggle with day sickness (hypersomnia).
> Your blood glucose level increases and with it the risk of being overweight and developing diabetes.
> Your immune system is weakened, and there are not enough defense mechanisms to protect the body from influenza viruses.
> Your performance and concentration are reduced.
> Your cortisol (stress hormone) level is constantly high, and you feel in continuous stress.
> You feel irritable and are subject to mood swings, which in the worst cases can lead to depression.

Chronotherapy: Back to the Circadian Rhythm

With circadian rhythm disturbances such as jet lag, shift work, or the backward-moving sleep phase syndrome, enough melatonin is produced but at the wrong time. Therefore, the use of melatonin in a timely manner and pulsatile-release are ways to restore the natural circadian rhythm.

This form of therapy is also called chronotherapy because it does not replace melatonin but rather regulates the endogenous release. The aforementioned melatonin analogs can also be used for this purpose.

Depending on the nature of the rhythm disturbance, the exact time of ingestion of melatonin should be chosen. The rule of thumb is that a dose between 6 p.m. and midnight shifts the rhythm forward. An intake after 2 a.m. shifts the rhythm backward (that is, to the previous day).

Exogenous Sleep Disorders

Sleep disorders can have many causes. Some may occur as a result of malfunctions of the body, which are then referred to as endogenous sleep disturbances. Others are caused by external (exogenous) factors. Those can be divided as follows:

Jet Lag and Shift Work

Jet lag refers to the fact that in a short time, several time zones are passed, and the natural internal clock is no longer in line with the actual time. As a result, the hormone releases that are subject to a typical daily rhythm are mixed up. Jet lag increases as more time zones are crossed, since an adaptation of the inner rhythms only takes place slowly. Shift workers also have to deal with a disturbed day-night rhythm and all its side effects: they must constantly adapt themselves to a new sleep-wake rhythm—a heavy burden for their own bodies.

Typical symptoms of a disturbed sleep-wake rhythm through jet lag or shift work include nighttime insomnia, drowsiness during the day, general malaise, and other somatic symptoms, such as concentration and cardiovascular problems. Potential health effects are daily fatigue, problems falling or staying asleep, limited physical fitness, reduced thinking, mood swings, depression, gastrointestinal and psychosomatic problems, and reduced reaction time. In the worst case, cardiovascular disease, diabetes, and cancer develop.

Here, melatonin is effective in regulating the shifts of the sleep-wake rhythm, which occur particularly in flights over several time zones. Several studies have shown that melatonin accelerates the readaptation to the new time zone. It has also proven its worth in mitigating the other jet lag symptoms. There is, further, a melatonin therapy for shift workers, who often suffer from insomnia due to a change in their daily rhythm.

It is important that the exact time of administration be observed so that melatonin can activate the phase shift. An ideal time would be between 10 and 11 p.m. of the new time zone to treat jet lag, or approximately one hour before the new rest phase for shift workers. This type of chronotherapy can be supported by light therapy. This is best done in the morning of the new time zone for jet lag or immediately before the active phase with shift workers.

Pharmacologically Induced Sleep Disorders

Many medicines and beverages can also adversely affect melatonin output. For example, it has been demonstrated that certain sleeping pills, such as benzodiazepines, and heart medications, such as beta-blockers, suppress the production of melatonin.

One study showed that patients taking beta-blockers could be helped by the additional administration of melatonin to improve their sleep (Scheer et al. 2012). Excessive alcohol and caffeine consumption (e.g., coffee or black tea) has a negative effect on the circadian rhythm and the release of melatonin and thus produces sleep disturbances or unhealthy sleep.

Caution, Caffeine!

Recently, a study found that caffeine, especially when consumed at night, has a particularly dramatic effect on our circadian rhythm. A single cup of coffee or tea can delay the release of melatonin, and thus sleep, by up to an hour. As a consequence, the internal clock is clearly set back, and it is difficult to get up the next day (Burke et al. 2015).

Endogenous Sleep Disorders

In the case of endogenous sleep disturbances, either too little melatonin is produced in the body or melatonin is released at the wrong time, even though one is in the normal day-night rhythm. More than 50 percent of all sleep disorders are due to endogenous causes.

Reversed Sleep Onset Syndrome

When the sleep phase syndrome is reversed, there is a sleep disorder caused by a shifted melatonin rhythm. It is common in adolescents and younger adults who are often classified as "night owls." They make the night a day, stay awake until the early hours of the morning, and sleep until the afternoon.

If these people can follow their own sleep patterns, for example during the weekend, they are rested and active during the rest of the day. It is difficult if the everyday life of the affected person "interferes" with their physical rhythm and they have to

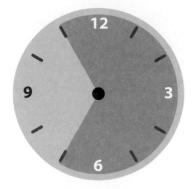
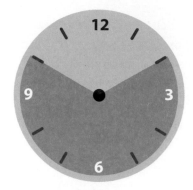

Normal sleep rhythm:
The person goes to bed at 11:00 p.m.
and gets up at 7:00 a.m.

Delayed sleep rhythm:
The person goes to bed at 2:00 a.m.
and gets up at 10:00 a.m.

Fig. 15: Pre- and postsleep phases.

get up again after a few hours of sleep in order to go to work or to school (see Fig. 15).

Scientists have been dealing with this rhythmic disorder for a long time, and all conclude that melatonin is most effective in treating this type of sleep disorder (Nagtegaal et al. 1998, Mundey et al. 2005).

Therapeutic Approach

The reversed sleep phase syndrome can be treated well with a chronotherapeutic approach in combination with a light therapy. What is important is to restore the rhythm. It is advisable to carry out light therapy early in the morning to shift the sleep-wake rhythm forward. Similar effects can be achieved by taking melatonin in the first hours of the evening, whether it is fast release or pulsatile.

Sleep-Wake Disorder in the Blind (Non-24 Syndrome)

Non-24 syndrome is a serious and chronic disorder of the day-night rhythm that occurs mainly in blind people. People who suffer from this disturbance of the 24-hour waking rhythm are not able to adjust their internal clock to the 24-hour rhythm of a day or to synchronize with it. These people live with their own rhythm, which is about 24.5–25 hours. This results in a tendency to fall asleep and wake up thirty minutes later. All other body rhythms, such as the body temperature, the hormone distribution, and the activity level, also shift accordingly.

Those affected have difficulty falling asleep during the night and are sleepy during the day. As with shift workers, they also struggle with a permanent change in their rhythm. There is no cure for the patients, but a perfectly coordinated melatonin therapy can help these people restore their rhythm and find a healthy sleep (Skene and Arendt 2007). This is the conclusion of a recently published study, which recommends a combined light and melatonin therapy to treat people who are suffering from non-24 syndrome to a controlled sleep-wake rhythm (Uchiyama and Lockley 2015). However, this combination is helpful only in those patients who still have the receptors in the retina that are responsible for the recognition of light.

Therapeutic Approach

The aim of a chronobiologically correct therapy is to synchronize the internal clock of those people with the normal 24-hour rhythm of the day. For this purpose, a morning light therapy can be used, under certain conditions, as well as substances that suppress daytime fatigue. However, this only works with those who are still minimally able to perceive light and dark. On the other hand, in all other patients, the evening dose of melatonin or similar drugs should not only stimulate sleep at night, but also serve as a timer to adjust the internal clock.

In order to adjust the body rhythm of blind people to the normal day-night rhythm, various substances can be used.

Alternatively, melatonin can be administered as a timer hormone in the evening. When the patient takes melatonin, whether it is a fast-release formula or a pulsatile one, the body is given a signal that tells it that it is now night. Recently, there have also been melatonin-like substances, such as tasimelteon or other analogs, which also have to be taken in the evening to set the internal clock to a normal day-night rhythm via the melatonin receptors in the brain.

Sleep Disorders in Old Age and in Special Living Conditions

Although its life-prolonging effect has not yet been demonstrated in humans, it is clear that melatonin has an extremely positive effect on the quality of life, particularly in old age. Thus, the hormone appears to be effective in the treatment of various processes associated with aging, such as disturbances of sleep-wake rhythm, hypertension, and deficits in the immune system. Presumably, the hormone is also helpful in delaying cell loss and deterioration of the body—factors that contribute to the aging process.

Due to the age-related decline in the nocturnal melatonin level, elderly people often suffer from sleep disturbances. At present, it is estimated that about one in two people over 65 are affected by this age-related sleep disorder. Here, treatment with melatonin proved to be helpful.

A study has investigated the levels of melatonin in people over 65 years and concluded that nocturnal melatonin concentration can decrease markedly as age progresses. The study's authors recommend that this be taken into account when taking additional medication (Scholtens et al. 2016).

Studies also showed that the use of melatonin not only caused improved sleep quality, but also decreased depression and anxiety. The positive effect of the hormone could be due to its ability to normalize the circadian rhythm. Such a regenerated rhythm influences all other physiological processes and contributes significantly to the improvement of the quality of life.

Menopause

Menopause is accompanied by profound hormonal changes, which not only lead to sleep problems, but also to other symptoms. The extent to which melatonin secretion also changes is still the subject of investigations. However, studies on women in menopause showed that the function of their thyroid gland improved when they took melatonin (Jehan et al. 2015). In addition, most women who were treated with melatonin reported a generally improved mood and a clear lessening of depression. This thesis is supported by the fact that high melatonin concentrations improve the general well-being in old age and lead to a reduced incidence of old-age types of diseases.

One study even showed that there was a correlation between a disturbed circadian rhythm in women in menopause and a decreased bone density (Wang et al. 2015). Another work confirmed that insomnia in women in menopause increases their risk of injury drastically (Zaslavsky et al. 2015).

Disturbed Sleep in Atopic Dermatitis

Sleep disturbances often also affect people who are suffering from neurodermatitis. Itching, especially in the evening and at night, is a typical symptom of this skin disease. The deprivation of sleep exacerbates suffering, but after a troubled night, those affected have to fight with the consequences of sleep deprivation. A study investigated children suffering from neurodermatitis and sleep disturbances and concluded that melatonin can alleviate their sleep problems and the severity of their disease at night (Chang et al. 2016b).

Melatonin Helps Cancer Patients with Sleep Disorders

Even cancer patients who often suffer from insomnia can be helped with a melatonin regimen, per the results of an Indian study. For this study, fifty volunteers aged twenty to sixty-five were given melatonin for fourteen days in the evening. As a result, not only did the drowsiness of the affected people decrease, but their sleep itself also significantly improved. Therefore, the researchers of this study recommend a daily dose of melatonin two hours before bedtime in order to reduce or increase the sleep-in phase and the sleep quality of cancer patients (Kurdi and Muthukalai 2016).

Neuropsychiatric Disorders

Our mental health is a complex system. Biological, psychological, and social factors play important roles in psychiatric diseases, and unfortunately, they are on the rise. The WHO estimates that depression will be the second most common disease by 2030. Studies suggest that a disturbed circadian rhythm could be responsible for many mental disorders, from clinical depression to bipolar disorder (Karatsoreos 2014).

Rhythm Disorders

What is common to most neuropsychiatric disorders, such as depression, Alzheimer's disease, and Parkinson's disease, is a day-night rhythm that seems to be completely out of step. Patients suffer from severe fatigue during the day and sleep problems at night. The elderly are affected more than all others, as their melatonin level is either too low or has shifted. One study recently showed that a regimen that restores the circadian rhythm through more sunlight during the day, a complementary melatonin input in the evening, and varied social and physical activities helps people alleviate their suffering (Abbott and Zee 2015).

Alzheimer's Disease

Alzheimer's disease is a progressive, neurodegenerative disease that typically affects memory, language, orientation, personality, and judgment. Disease symptoms manifest differently among people affected but have one thing in common: they become increasingly worse over time.

The causes of Alzheimer's disease are not clear. Genetic influences, such as heredity, seem to play a role, as well as risk factors for diabetes, increased cholesterol, hypertension, chronic stress, excess weight, and alcohol abuse.

Low Melatonin Levels in Alzheimer's Patients

Studies have shown that melatonin levels are significantly lower in Alzheimer's patients than in healthy people. It is therefore assumed that this hormone could play an important role in its treatment (Savaskan et al. 2005). In addition, studies in Alzheimer's patients have shown that those affected also have lower tryptophan and serotonin levels, which play important roles in the production of melatonin (Rosales-Corral et al. 2012).

Many studies have focused on the use of melatonin and how this can improve some symptoms of Alzheimer's, such as dementia or delirium. What also benefits the patient is that melatonin has no side effects, which is not the case with antipsychotics and sedatives (Alagiakrishnan 2016).

Sundowning

The unrest that many people with Alzheimer's and dementia suffer from is referred to as "sundowning." When the sun is lower, as in the late afternoon hours, the prolonged shadows can confuse patients. They often react with roaming, screaming, or aggressive behavior. This can be a difficult and dangerous situation not only for the patients, who often hurt themselves during these times, but also for their relatives and caretakers.

Sundowning is associated with a disturbance of the circadian rhythm, as the sleep-wake rhythm of the Alzheimer's patients is reversed. They are cheerful and awake during the night, but sleepy during the day (Klaffke and Staedt 2006). Some of them are very excited during the early evening or late afternoon, because they have not moved enough during the day as a result of their fatigue or have been, paradoxically, too active. A melatonin administration, parallel to a light therapy, could help these patients to regain their biological rhythm and to achieve a higher quality of life in their illness (Dowling et al. 2008).

Movement and Melatonin against Alzheimer's

In a study from 2012, Alzheimer's patients were treated with a combination of melatonin and physical exercise. This treatment reduced behavioral and psychological symptoms, such as anxiety and cognitive impairment. The oxidative stress in the brain, an important factor contributing to Alzheimer's, had also been reduced (García-Mesa et al. 2012).

Another study investigated the effect of a combined therapy of bright light in the morning and oral intake of melatonin in the evening. This therapy is quite effective in improving the waking phases and the activity of Alzheimer's patients housed in inpatient facilities (Dowling et al. 2008). Some researchers have also reported that music therapy increases melatonin secretion, a therapeutic approach that is also used in therapy for Alzheimer's (Kumar et al. 1999).

Parkinson's

Parkinson's disease is one of the most common neurodegenerative diseases for which there is no cure. It is caused by the fact that certain brain neurons lose the ability to produce dopamine, a neurotransmitter that supports cognitive function, emotional control, movement coordination, and a variety of other important functions in our body.

What is Dopamine?

Dopamine is a neurotransmitter that is regarded as a happiness hormone, much like serotonin. It is primarily responsible for our mood, attention, ability to learn, and motor activities, as well as sleep.

The symptoms of Parkinson's disease begin slowly, and the disease continues to develop slowly for years. If the diagnosis is made, 70 percent of the dopamine-producing neurons are often already dead. This makes the effective treatment of Parkinson's very difficult (Mahmood et al. 2016).

The lack of dopamine impairs a variety of physical functions, typically causing slow muscle movements, tremors, or muscle stiffness. Sleep problems and loss of the sense of smell (anosmia) also usually accompany the disease.

Melatonin in Parkinson's Disease

Although Parkinson's disease is primarily associated with the decrease of dopamine in the brain, melatonin also appears to play a role. This could explain the connection with sleep disorders. While Parkinson's disease progresses, melatonin production decreases in the brain (Breen et al. 2016).

Periodically taking melatonin can help people with Parkinson's sleep and protect their brain from further degenerative changes. Several studies suggest that the stabilization of sleep cycles by taking melatonin should be a standard part of the disease treatment (Srinivasan et al. 2011).

Some research also demonstrates a link between sleep disorders and the development of Parkinson's disease. A new study suggests that a treated or regulated sleep-wake disorder in the early stages of Parkinson's disease can delay those symptoms that affect motor function and movement for years. This makes it possible for those affected to live longer and healthier lives (Lauretti et al. 2016).

A recent study showed that melatonin, in addition to improving sleep disorders, also has a positive effect on anxiety disorders, depression, memory disorders, as well as on motor disorders typical in Parkinsonian patients (Mack et al. 2016).

People with Parkinson's who take melatonin show fewer and weaker symptoms than those who do not. For a long time, this was attributed to the healing nature of sufficient sleep. But today, we know that melatonin is not only a sleep-inducing hormone, but also a neuroprotective one. Melatonin can reduce, sometimes even prevent, the loss of the nerve cells and thus damage to the brain, as well as support the cells during their regeneration (Gutierrez-Valdez et al. 2012, Yildirim et al. 2014).

Epilepsy

Epilepsy is a disturbance of the electrical conductivity of the nerve cells in the brain. Those affected suffer from convulsions or temporary unconsciousness. Other forms of epilepsy are caused by oxidative stress (e.g., free radicals) or high fever.

Years ago, researchers discovered that seizures usually have a 24-hour rhythm and have established a connection with the circadian melatonin secretion. The effect of melatonin on the seizures was examined in tests, with the result that the frequency of certain epileptic seizures decreased (Fauteck et al. 1995).

Sleep Disorders and Epilepsy

Studies have repeatedly found a link between sleep disorders and epilepsy, which in turn suggests that the circadian rhythm has an impact on the onset of seizures (Quigg 2000, Manni et al. 2016). A brief sleep deprivation, even for just one night, is used to detect epileptic seizures better in the EEG. A recent study of epileptic children between the ages of six and eleven found that the children's sleep improved with the intake of melatonin (Jain et al. 2015). In one study, melatonin helped children with their sleep disorders and the severity and frequency of their seizures (Fauteck et al. 1999).

Melatonin Can Relieve Symptoms

Further studies with children confirmed that the administration of melatonin reduced the severity and frequency of epileptic seizures (Guo and Yao 2009). The hormone can act as a neuroprotector against oxidative stress due to its antioxidant properties in the central nervous system, which is particularly evident in patients with epilepsy.

In addition, specific melatonin receptors could be detected on the cerebral cortex, whose stimulation by melatonin suppresses the formation of an attack (Fauteck et al. 1999a). Thus, melatonin with different mechanisms of action seems to have a positive effect on a variety of different epilepsy forms, with regard to both the development and the severity of seizures (Lima et al. 2011).

Good Success with Chronotherapy

Chronotherapeutic treatment, meaning an individual, time-oriented medication, can achieve very good results in people with epilepsy (Stanley et al. 2014).

In addition to chronopharmacology, other forms of chronotherapy can also be used to treat epilepsy patients. One example is light therapy, which corrects circadian imbalances and can help to alleviate some symptoms of epilepsy. On the other hand, short, constantly repeated light pulses can trigger a seizure—an effect that is also used for the diagnosis of epilepsy.

Attention-Deficit/Hyperactivity Disorder

Attention-deficit/hyperactivity disorder (ADHD), among the most common psychological disorders in children and adolescents, is characterized by problems with attention, self-regulation, and impulsiveness, as well as a physical restlessness (hyperactivity). Children who suffer from ADHD cannot sit still, do not listen, and always want to have things go their way.

Adults may also be affected by ADHD, but with the exception of attention deficit disorder, symptoms are different (e.g., depression, anxiety, and eating disorders). The causes of ADHD have not yet been fully explored. It is assumed that genetics play a role, as well as a lack of dopamine.

Melatonin Helps Children with ADHD

Sleep disorders are widespread in children who suffer from ADHD. A recent study investigated the long-term intake of melatonin and its effect on children with ADHD. According to parents, 88 percent of the children treated showed a reduction in their sleep problems. In addition, 71 percent reported an improvement in day-to-day behavior, and 61 percent reported an improvement in mood (Hoebert et al. 2009).

Schizophrenia

Schizophrenia is one of the most serious and debilitating neuropsychiatric disorders. Symptoms include hallucinations, emotional disorders, and decreased motor skills. Researchers are intensively trying to find medicines that enable those affected to live normal lives.

The exact causes of schizophrenia are still unknown. A number of factors are believed to influence this serious disease, including a disorder of neurotransmitters, the messenger in the brain that normally transmit signals to the nerve cells. Studies on patients also detected changes in their brains themselves. Genetic inheritance appears to play an essential role in schizophrenia.

Disturbed Sleep-Wake Rhythm

Schizophrenia is another neuropsychiatric disorder found to be associated with disturbed circadian rhythms and decreasing melatonin levels. It is therefore assumed that melatonin could help in the treatment of the disease. In addition, the hormone could increase the effect of antipsychotic drugs and reduce their side effects.

Many chronobiological studies conclude that a disturbance of the circadian rhythm may be partly responsible for the effects of this physical disorder (Wulff et al. 2012).

A study with patients of schizophrenia used melatonin in combination with a popular antipsychotic drug. Another patient group who participated in the same study also received this drug, but instead of melatonin, a placebo was administered. Those who received melatonin experienced fewer side effects, such as weight gain and a lower PANSS, a value that measures the severity of schizophrenia symptoms (Baandrup et al. 2017).

Depression

Depression is a disease that occurs with higher frequency now than ever before; it is characterized by symptoms such as lack of energy, hopelessness, negative thoughts, sleep disorders and, in the worst cases, suicidal thoughts. Depression also manifests itself physically, for example, sleepiness during the daytime, sleeplessness during the nighttime, muscle pain, gastrointestinal discomfort, and headaches.

Serotonin Deficiency

People suffering from depression almost always have a functional disorder of their serotonin level. You will remember that serotonin is one of the most important neurotransmitters (messenger substances) in the human body and is also often referred to as a happiness hormone because our mental well-being is largely influenced by our serotonin level.

Serotonin deficiency, especially in the brain, reduces our mood and creates a bad state of mind. As serotonin is also responsible for the development of melatonin in the evening, serotonin deficiency can lead to insomnia.

Melatonin Relieves Symptoms of Depression

There are studies that show melatonin can improve at least some symptoms of depression, especially those related to sleep (see, for example, Kunz 2012). Patients with severe depression were treated with melatonin, which was effective in improving the subjective sleep quality of those affected. In addition, positive effects were found for patients suffering from seasonal depression. In combination with conventional drugs for depression, melatonin can increase antidepressant effectiveness even further (Hirsch-Rodriguez et al. 2007).

Another study reported reduced depression in patients with SAD who were treated with low-dose melatonin in the afternoon. A small dose of melatonin improved the synchronization of the internal clock and the biological day rhythm with the altered light conditions prevailing in the winter (Meliska et al. 2013). In this case, it is a classical chronotherapeutic approach.

Another study establishes a connection between circadian rhythm and nutrition. The brain appears particularly sensitive to metabolic events, depending on the light-dark cycle (Leheste and Torres 2015). This seems to contribute to the fact that depressive people often have a disturbed eating habit.

Seasonal Affective Disorder (SAD)

SAD is a specific form of depression that occurs mainly in the autumn and winter months. The primary symptoms are a depressed mood, a reduction in the levels of energy, anxiety, a longer duration of sleep, an increased appetite for carbohydrates, and weight gain. In the case of seasonally independent depression, appetite loss, weight loss, and sleep shortage occur.

As SAD has been described more often in regions where very long nights prevail in the wintertime (such as the polar regions), people who live there are now believed to suffer from a disturbed melatonin production. In these individuals, more melatonin was released over a longer period of time but was mostly delayed.

Melatonin and Light

Even a small, early evening dose of melatonin in a fast-release dosage form improves the consistency of the internal clock and the biological daily rhythm during the winter so that mood improves significantly. Light therapy has also proven to be a useful form of treatment. Used in the morning, the light not only reduces the morning melatonin, but also improves the entire rhythm.

Melatonin as a Supplement

Recent studies in chronobiology have shown that melatonin supplements can help treat circadian sleep disorders and solve a variety of sleep-related problems. However, not all melatonin supplements are the same. The way melatonin is released from these supplements can have an enormous impact on the physiological values and effects of this hormone.

Some people report that melatonin does not work as drastically as they would have expected. They often assume that melatonin is not useful in treating their sleep problems when in fact they have simply chosen the wrong type of melatonin supplement. It should also be noted that melatonin does not act as a classic hypnotic, but as a regulator of the sleep-wake rhythm. Hence, the effect is most accurately assessed when one is asked in the morning how restful their sleep was—and not how long it took to fall asleep or how often one woke up.

Slow or Fast Release

Most melatonin preparations have either a fast or a slow release of the hormone. A rapid release of melatonin leads to a steep increase in melatonin levels, which falls again after one to two hours. People who take this type of supplement find that they become drowsy quickly but have difficulty sleeping or simply fail to get quality sleep.

Slowly released melatonin, on the other hand, takes hours to induce sleep and often does not decrease in the early morning hours. People who choose preparations that allow a slow release of melatonin may have problems with falling asleep due to the initial low melatonin level, followed by difficulties waking up, as the morning values are still unnaturally high.

Timed Release

A timed release of melatonin is a supplement designed to release the hormone exactly in the amount that mimics a healthy natural melatonin level. It is released stepwise so that the melatonin level increases rapidly after the supplement has been taken and then remains at a high level for several hours. The values then fall off again quickly in the morning to allow a wake up. This mimics healthy, normal circadian rhythm cycles, which are associated with restful sleep.

Research in the field of chronobiology has shown that the maintenance of melatonin cycles is important not only for restful sleep, but also for general health. For this reason, more and more health experts recommend the timed release of melatonin as an ideal supplement. Ensuring a healthy circadian rhythm is important to health; therefore, timed melatonin is usually the best option. Initial clinical examinations have shown that such dosage forms not only promote falling asleep and staying asleep, but also significantly improve sleep quality (Stankov et al. 2010, Kolev et al. 2011). (See Fig. 16.)

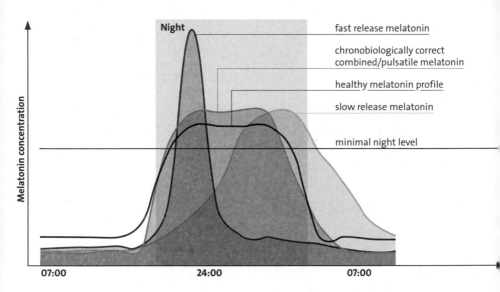

Fig. 16: Schematic representation of different dosage forms of melatonin preparations. The rapid-release form, the slow/sustained release, and the chronobiologically correct combined/pulsatile-release form, as well as the normal melatonin rhythm of an adult, are presented.

Headache

Each of us knows headaches and how much they can influence our well-being. Headaches can be caused by a myriad of events, including changes in weather or having spent too much time in front of a computer. Ideally, in most cases, the symptoms quickly disappear when we get some fresh air, take more breaks, and rest.

For many people, however, headaches have become an almost daily companion, which can become very bothersome and painful. The symptoms of a severe migraine can spread throughout the whole body: nausea, vomiting, severe fatigue, and high sensitivity to light and noise. It usually helps the affected person to stay in dark rooms in order to alleviate the discomfort, which in the worst case can last not only hours, but days.

For the many people affected, migraine drugs have a number of side effects, such as dizziness, irregular heartbeats, and diarrhea. These drugs can trigger a negative cycle for these people, making it impossible for them to pursue their usual everyday life during this time, and their quality of life is severely impaired.

Melatonin against Migraine

Numerous studies have shown that migraines can be successfully treated by melatonin. The exact mechanism is not known at the moment, but there are many connections between the circadian rhythm and this type of headache (Solomon 1992).

Most people who suffer from migraines get them at about the same time each day, suggesting a circadian component. An older study investigated the relationship between sleep disorders and migraine attacks and found that 79 percent of the migraine attacks among study participants were preceded by a sleepless night (Alstadhaug et al. 2007).

This could be due to a gene associated with circadian rhythm disturbances. It appears to be one of the main causes of this type of headache and concomitant sleep disorders. The use of melatonin provides a very positive double effect for patients suffering from both symptoms: it prevents migraines and simultaneously promotes a healthy sleep-wake cycle (Gelfand and Goadsby 2016).

Another recent study has shown that sleep quality can also affect the frequency of migraine attacks. Researchers observed that a group of poor sleepers suffered significantly more frequently from migraines than the comparison groups, which is an important finding for the pharmacological prevention of migraines (Lin et al. 2016).

And yet another recent study has shown that melatonin has an excellent effect in the prevention of migraine. Subjects were given 3 mg of melatonin, 25 g of amitriptyline (a common antimigraine agent), or a placebo administered for twelve weeks. The result: melatonin is as effective as amitriptyline and causes no side effects (Gonçalves et al. 2016a).

Cluster Headaches

Melatonin studies have also shown promise for treating so-called cluster headaches, which occur spontaneously. Cluster headaches are characterized by strong, one-sided headaches in the area of the eye and temple. Tearful eyes or a runny nose are typical symptoms. The pain reaches its maximum after about twenty minutes and will decrease after a few hours. The affected are often symptom-free until the attacks recur. In the worst case, they can last for weeks, usually with a few attacks daily.

As with migraines, researchers also linked cluster headaches to a disturbed sleep-wake rhythm and the pain attacks that occur (Barloese 2015).

Melatonin as an Effective Painkiller

This leads to the conclusion that a lack of melatonin can lead to nocturnal pain or even pain during the day. In some patients, the frequency of headaches was significantly reduced with the help of melatonin (Srinivasan et al. 2012).

There are many mechanisms that may be responsible for the positive effect of melatonin. On one hand, there is an anti-inflammatory effect. On the other hand, it inhibits the excessive release of dopamine, stabilizes the cell membrane, and promotes the release of GABA—the most important neurotransmitter of the brain. In addition, melatonin acts as a protector against free radicals and regulates the vascular nerves and thus the blood flow (Srinivasan et al. 2012).

Chronic Pain

Fibromyalgia (FMA) is a chronic pain disorder that affects approximately 4 percent of the population, women in particular. The word "fibromyalgia" is a combination of the Latin word "fibra" (fibrous) for fibrous connective tissue and the Greek words "myos" (muscle) and "algos" (pain). In fact, muscle, tendon, and ligament pain are all main symptoms of this disease.

Other symptoms include fatigue, depression, anxiety, insomnia, and morning stiffness. Some also experience cardiovascular disorders, balance impairment, and abnormal gastrointestinal activity. Patients also report a degradation of their memory and cognitive functions (Srinivasan et al. 2012).

Despite numerous studies, it has not yet been possible to establish clear causes of this chronic disease. Researchers assume, however, that messengers in the brain of those affected do not function as they do in healthy people. Studies have also shown that FMA patients have low serotonin and melatonin levels (Mahdi et al. 2011).

Melatonin: The Body-Borne Pain Medication

Numerous studies deal with the relationship between melatonin and pain. Findings suggest that melatonin is not only the hormone that helps guide our innate circadian rhythm and our biological twenty-four-hour clock, but also serves as a regulator for pain signals. The hormone acts indirectly on the so-called opioid receptors. These are the same receptors on which many painkillers act (Ambriz-Tututi et al. 2009; Danilov and Kurganova 2016).

Melatonin Improves FMS Symptoms

In fact, in a series of trials, the use of melatonin significantly improved a variety of FMA symptoms. Patients were given melatonin daily for six weeks. One group received melatonin alone, the other in combination with a conventional drug prescribed for FMA. In both groups, the symptoms improved significantly (Zanette et al. 2014).

These findings provide hope for many people living with FMA and other pain syndromes. Especially in the case of diseases of this kind, patients have been given opiates (very strong drugs for pain), which not only have unpleasant side effects, but are also addictive.

Eyes

The eye is our most important sensory organ, with which we perceive our environment and communicate external stimuli with functions in our body. All this takes place via light stimuli, primarily due to the difference between day and night. The photoreceptors play an important role. They pass the visual signals over nerve cells to our brain, which affects functions in all the organs in our body.

Melatonin Production in the Eye

Melatonin is produced not only in the pineal gland, but also in the retina. Melatonin has many important functions, including the control of the eye pigmentation and thus the regulation of the amount of light that reaches the photoreceptors of the eye. In addition, melatonin protects the outermost leaf of the retina, or retinal pigment epithelium, from oxidative damage.

Relationship between Ocular Diseases and Melatonin

The British Journal of Ophthalmology recently published an alarming relationship between aging eyes and melatonin production. Measurements show that after the age of 45, fewer sunrays reach the inner eye. This is the result of the slight yellowing of the eyepiece lens and the narrowing of the pupil. For this reason, fewer light particles reach the most important cells in the retina that measure the day-night rhythm to regulate our internal clock.

Studies show that changes in the aging eye lead to a series of typical eye diseases in which the cause cannot be found in the eye itself. The consequences of worsening visual power include cognitive deficits (especially memory capacity), insomnia, depression, and prolonged response times. A correlation between this change in the eye and a disturbed melatonin production is therefore always emphasized.

Macular Degeneration

This complex eye disease—also called age-related macular degeneration (AMD)—is one of the most frequent causes of blindness in adults. This affects the center of the retina, which is responsible for sharp vision and is destroyed over the course of the disease.

In addition to genetic causes, the well-known risk factors are age, hypertension, lifestyle (e.g., smoking and excess weight), sun, strong UV light, and oxidative stress (see Fig. 17).

Even if the exact correlation between genetic and environmental factors has not yet been clarified, scientists agree that oxidative stress plays an important role in the disease process of macular degeneration (Blasiak et al. 2016). People with dark eyes suffer less frequently from this eye disease.

Symptoms include a decrease in visual acuity and the ability to read. Patients have difficulty with contrast and color

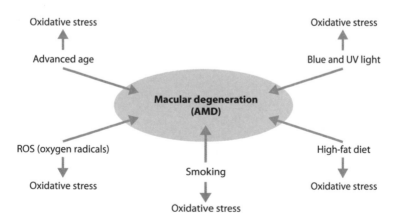

Fig. 17: Oxidative stress and other factors leading to macular degeneration (modified by Blasiak et al. 2016).

vision. They also react very sensitively to bright, dazzling lights and have difficulty adapting to changing light conditions. In the further course of the disease, central facial field failures occur; the patients can recognize people, but not their facial features.

Retina Follows Circadian Rhythm

It should not surprise you that your retina also has its own circadian rhythm. The "clock" genes in the eye ensure that important processes are regulated—including melatonin release or dopamine synthesis (Ruan et al. 2006). These genes are also involved in all processes that affect the function of photoreceptors.

Melatonin Protects as an Antioxidant

Recently, a study focused on the interplay of circadian rhythm, oxidative stress, and AMD (Fanjul-Moles and López-Riquelme 2016). Even if further studies are required, the results of this study showed that a disturbed circadian rhythm seems to contribute to degenerative processes in the retina that are responsible for the death of cells.

Melatonin with its high potency as an antioxidant can help to prevent the destruction of cells by free radicals and thus delay the progress of the disease and to protect the retina. Whether melatonin acts only as a radical scavenger or there are also receptor-mediated effects is still the subject of research.

Although there are still too few clinical trials to make a definitive, binding statement, some studies have already concluded that patients with macular degeneration have a melatonin deficiency (e.g., Rosen et al. 2012), which could be addressed with replacement therapy.

Glaucoma

Glaucoma (green star) is a conglomerate of different eye diseases, all of which lead to a loss of optic nerve fibers. The main cause of this disease is an increased pressure in the eye chamber, often coupled with low blood pressure in the vessels that supply the retina. A weak circulation of the optic nerve through a blockage of the blood vessels can also lead to glaucoma, as can chronic inflammation caused by an unhealthy lifestyle that favors oxidative stress, such as excessive UV light, smoking, and so forth.

If disease has progressed, the optic nerve may die, the external nerves being damaged first and then gradually the internal nerves. The result is the reduction of the visual field—from the outer edge to the inside—that can ultimately lead to complete blindness.

Melatonin, the Universal Talent

Research has shown that photoreceptors can also be lost by oxidative stress from glaucoma. Melatonin can be effective by reducing pressure in the eyes as well as protecting the photoreceptors from free radicals.

Precisely for the regulation of intraocular pressure, numerous studies with animals showed that melatonin can achieve outstanding effects (Martínez-Águila et al. 2016). It has also been shown that a melatonin deficiency is a high-risk factor for developing glaucoma (Tosini et al. 2013). All studies conclude that melatonin therapy is particularly useful for people who have a melatonin deficiency.

Cardiovascular Disease

Cardiovascular disease is one of the most frequent causes of death, at around 45 percent worldwide. Medical professionals expect this figure will rise in the coming years (Griebler et al. 2014).

Hypertension, myocardial infarction, and stroke are all illnesses with a common denominator: blood can no longer flow unimpeded. Important organs, such as the heart and brain, are therefore not adequately supplied.

Rhythmic Cardiovascular Functions

Our cardiovascular system also follows the circadian rhythm. Shortly before we wake up, our body increasingly pours out the hormones we need to go from sleep to waking. In doing so, our blood pressure and pulse rate increase, so that we can get fit and active in the day. If we are healthy, this process is completely normal for our bodies.

However, for people with heart disease, the rapid rise of these hormones can be a health hazard. Increased blood pressure and the task of pumping even more blood are big burdens for the heart. Heart attacks are therefore more frequent in the morning, as are strokes.

Disturbance and Risk Factors for our Cardiovascular System

Age, stress, smoking, alcohol, fatty food, exercise deficit, excess weight, and diabetes mellitus are all factors that contribute to our cardiovascular system not functioning as it should.

The influence of our lifestyle on heart health should not be underestimated! For example, longer-lasting stress can lead to a deficiency of blood circulation in the coronary arteries and in the worst case even cause a heart attack. Above all, stress hormones, which increase the blood pressure and the heart rate considerably, are shed. The risk of diseases of the cardiovascular system such as arteriosclerosis, hypertension, coronary heart disease, and myocardial infarction increases dramatically.

High Blood Pressure

High blood pressure (hypertension) is one of the most common diseases in many western cultures. The pressure in the vessels is increased to ensure that sufficient blood flow through narrowed vessels. This high pressure can promote vascular constriction, which can lead to stroke, myocardial infarction, and other vascular diseases.

The circadian rhythm is particularly noticeable in the case of blood pressure. It reaches its peak in the morning, then declines during the day until it is at its lowest between midnight and 3 a.m. Our pulse also follows this rhythm.

Melatonin Regulates Blood Pressure

Melatonin has been shown to be effective in the regulation of blood pressure. Studies in Pechanova et al. 2014 have shown that the oral administration of melatonin reduces both high blood pressure and associated vascular reactivity. This effect results from the fact that the hormone has a relaxing effect on the vessels and acts as a potent free radical scavenger, since these free radicals have a negative influence on blood pressure (Sánchez-Barceló et al. 2010).

Above all, long-term melatonin therapy showed very positive effects on subjects in several studies. Their nocturnal hypertension could be successfully regulated and reduced (e.g., Scheer et al. 2004, Cagnacci et al. 2005). However, it has not yet been possible to clarify exactly how these mechanisms of melatonin affect blood pressure, even if there are different theories.

Arteriosclerosis

It develops slowly, over decades—mostly without conspicuous symptoms. Arteriosclerosis is the cause of narrowed or closed blood vessels in over 90 percent of patients with chronic circulatory problems.

The vessel walls become calcified, as a result of which the vessel diameter becomes narrower, and the blood can no longer flow freely to the organs. Consequently, blood pressure increases, and vital organs are often no longer sufficiently supplied with blood—a serious undersupply with serious consequences. The risk of a heart attack or a stroke increases rapidly as a result of this arterial calcification.

Heart Attack

In the case of a heart attack, an acute vascular occlusion occurs. The tissue supplied by this vessel suffers from an oxygen deficiency and is damaged.

The primary goal of therapy is, therefore, to restore the blood or oxygen supply within a very short amount of time. However, as soon as the oxygen supply necessary for life returns, further oxidative damage occurs to the already-attacked tissue due to the influx of oxygen. This is referred to as a reperfusion injury.

Melatonin Reduces Cell Damage

These damages can be significantly mitigated, if not prevented, by administering higher doses of melatonin. Early studies show that melatonin can significantly reduce the extent of cell damage in these situations thanks to its antioxidant and anti-inflammatory effect (Pei et al. 2016, Ozsoy et al. 2016). In order to achieve this effect, though, melatonin must be given immediately after the occlusion of the vessel, irrespective of the time of day.

Melatonin for Your Cardiovascular Health

Melatonin is one of the most effective antioxidants in our body. It protects our heart and vessels from harmful cholesterol deposits. It also reduces stress hormones, lowers blood pressure, and thus has an immensely positive effect on our cardiovascular system.

Melatonin could also be useful in reducing cardiac hypertrophy, particularly to the cardiac region, thereby reducing the incidence of heart attacks. The hormone also acts as an opponent of free radicals that attack the heart muscle. Since melatonin also has anti-inflammatory properties, it could be used effectively in treating arteriosclerosis. Some in vitro studies have shown that melatonin is efficient in the inhibition of LDL oxidation. In simplified terms, the deposition of cholesterol on vessel walls is reduced, which is regarded as one of the main causes of arteriosclerosis. In order to have this effect in your own body, scientists advise that melatonin be taken as a precautionary measure in the evening.

Stroke

Stroke is the second most common cause of death worldwide (Andrabi et al. 2015). According to the Centers for Disease Control, in the United States alone, 130,000 people a year die from this circulatory disturbance of the brain, and more than 795,000 have a stroke. Those affected often suffer the consequences for many years with lengthy rehab stays. A stroke often causes the loss of cognitive abilities, which is called vascular (or vascular-related) dementia (Kalaria 2012). Our brain is a very complex organ that controls important functions in our body. Any small disturbance can, therefore, have serious consequences for our health.

What Happens During a Stroke?

If the brain is not adequately supplied with blood, a stroke can occur. In the majority of cases (approximately 85 percent), the cause is a blocked vessel in the brain, which leads to an oxygen deficiency in the respective brain region. The nearby nerve cells die and affect the function of the area. For example, those affected may experience speech or visual disturbances, suffer paralysis symptoms, or might no longer be able to lift an arm. This is also known as an ischemic injury. The calcification of the arteries, as is the case with arteriosclerosis, is due to the blockage of the vessel. In the remaining 15 percent of all strokes, the sudden bursting of a vessel is the cause of stroke, inducing hemorrhagic injury or cerebral hemorrhage. In this case, too, the downstream tissue is no longer adequately supplied and dies off slowly.

Risk Factors for Stroke

The risk factors for stroke such as high blood pressure, high cholesterol, diabetes, or excess weight, as well as too much alcohol, smoking, and lack of exercise, can be reduced—as can be the factors affecting lifestyle.

Many studies have shown that shift work is one of the risk factors that favor a stroke. Recently, a study showed that shift work could adversely affect the severity of a stroke, especially in men (Earnest et al. 2016). Studies have shown years ago that the relationship among hypertension, vascular function, and the circadian clock is a key factor in the development of stroke (Rudic 2009). If you are constantly exposed to a change of the day-waking rhythm, as is the case with shift workers, you must expect an increased risk of a stroke.

Oxidative Stress

Our central nervous system is extremely susceptible to oxidative stress for many reasons. On the one hand, the brain interacts with the oxygen we inhale. With each breath, however, the risk of free radicals also increases. In addition, our brains have a small number of body-borne antioxidants, and some acids in our brains support these oxidation processes (Watson et al. 2016). It is precisely oxidative stress that can adversely affect the severity of a stroke.

Melatonin Protects the Brain

Numerous studies have shown that melatonin has a positive effect not just in prevention (Pei et al. 2002), but also in acute stroke treatment (Watson et al. 2016). Its antioxidative potency is often documented and could significantly help in the event of stroke in order to alleviate further damage in the brain (Andrabi et al. 2015). In order to prevent a stroke, melatonin should be taken long-term in the evening. When the stroke has occurred, it is important to immediately give higher doses of melatonin, as in myocardial infarction, regardless of the time of day.

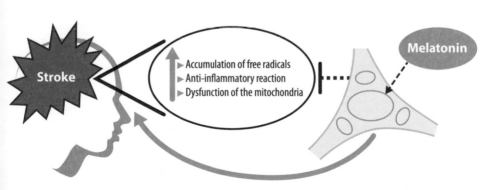

Figure 18: Protective effect of melatonin in stroke
(modified according to Watson et al. 2016).

Digestive System

The digestive organs are an important part of our physical and emotional health. We understand all the organs and glands involved in the uptake, processing, and transport of food. This starts with the mouth and throat, via the esophagus, pancreas, liver, and gall bladder, to the gastrointestinal tract, the largest part of our digestive system.

Digestion is mainly monitored and maintained by the parasympathetic and sympathetic nervous systems, which are collectively referred to as the autonomous nervous system. While the sympathetic supports the performance of our body, the parasympathetic provides rest and recovery of our organs and stimulates our metabolism and thus our entire digestive system.

Studies have shown that the parasympathetic nervous system, which stimulates the body to digest food, is most active in non-REM sleep. The sympathetic nervous system, which slows down digestion, changes during REM sleep with the parasympathetic. This balance and interplay of the autonomic nervous system are incredibly important to maintain good bowel health (Vaughn et al. 2014).

Increased Melatonin Production in the Digestive Tract

The cells in the digestive tract produce four hundred times as much melatonin as the pineal gland. However, this melatonin is not primarily released into the blood, but presumably acts directly on the spot. It, therefore, does not have the characteristic of a timer, as melatonin produced in the pineal gland during the night does.

Although the exact function of melatonin in the digestive tract is not yet known, melatonin protects against ulcers of the gastric mucosa thanks to its antioxidant properties. Whether receptor-mediated mechanisms of action play a role here is still the subject of intensive research, but very probable.

Scientists have already found out that bacteria in our gut reacts to melatonin. They also follow a circadian rhythm adapted to our natural rhythm. As soon as the bacteria notice that melatonin is multiplied, they begin to heat up and become active. What exactly this behavior means is not yet known. However, what is certain is that the intestinal microbes react to our sleep-wake cycles and thus definitely change their behavior (Paulose et al. 2016)

Hormones Control Digestion

Many hormones that are associated with eating habits and digestion, such as ghrelin, insulin, and leptin, are produced cyclically over a twenty-four-hour period at very specific times. If no light is present for an extended period of time, these hormone cycles stop and are only randomly secreted.

Because these hormones can have a destructive effect in the gastrointestinal tract without eating, for example, when they trigger the additional production of stomach acid, this could be a cause of many gastrointestinal and nutritional disorders (Vaughn et al. 2014).

Gastroesophageal Reflux Disease

Almost every one of us has experienced heartburn or acid regurgitation. After too much, too fatty, too salty, or too acidic food, the burping leads to a painful burning, which can radiate from the stomach to the neck.

These complaints are caused by malfunctions of the lower esophageal sphincter. It usually ensures that the food tube close after swallowing the food. Incorrect eating behavior can lead to this small valve not being completely closed. It starts leaking, and the stomach acid comes in contact with the mucosa of the esophagus, causing the painful burning sensation.

Connection between Sleep and Heartburn

Have you ever woken up because of burning stomach acid, or has it prevented you from falling asleep? The flat lying position makes it impossible to fall asleep, and the symptoms seem endless.

Scientists have long ago discovered that there is a direct link among the circadian rhythm, sleep, and the nocturnal reflux. Studies in the area of circadian biology show that disturbances of the sleep-wake cycles can lead to heartburn, associated mucus damage, and stomach ulcers. One factor that might explain this is that gastric acid, stimulated by the parasympathetic, is formed at night in higher amounts. The consequence is that the burping and pain rob us of our sleep.

Melatonin Protects the Mucosa

In the case of gastroesophageal reflux syndrome, in which increased gastric acid is pushed into the esophagus, melatonin significantly reduces the oxidative damage of the mucous membrane and thus also the pain symptoms. Scientists suspect that melatonin serves as universal protection of the stomach lining from the salicylic acid that is contained not only in many foodstuffs, but also in anti-inflammatory and fever-reducing painkillers and for protection against *Helicobacter* bacteria—which play a superordinate and disease-causing role in gastritis (Vaughn et al. 2014).

Irritable Bowel

Unexplained abdominal pain, flatulence, altered stool habits such as constipation, diarrhea, and general malaise—each of us probably knows one or more such discomforts, which usually disappear, from time to time. However, for some people (or up to 15 percent of Americans), they become a daily burden that substantially affect quality of life. If the symptoms persist for more than three months, it is called irritable bowel syndrome.

Causes of Irritable Bowel Syndrome

How an irritable bowel syndrome starts and what is happening have not yet been fully investigated, mainly because each type of irritable bowel can have different causes. However, it is proven that diet and stress significantly influence the intestine and its activity. In addition, some drugs, such as antibiotics, can affect intestinal activity. In some people, the peristaltic function (mobility of the intestinal wall), which is particularly important for the removal of gases, is slowed or increased.

Still others react to the processes in the intestine with a lot of pain. For example, an affected person can acutely feel how the bowel expands during emptying. This is due to a larger number of nerve cells in the intestinal mucosa of the patients than is the case with other people. Serotonin, which controls intestinal motion and pain sensitivity, can also play a role.

Serotonin Controls Brain-Intestinal Axis

Researchers have found that there is a connection between the brain and the intestine. One speaks here of the brain-intestine axis (Carabotti et al. 2015). This axis allows our intestines and the bacteria that live there to influence our health in many ways. For example, people with an imbalance of gut flora tend to suffer from PTSD, that is, post-traumatic stress disorder. The exact mechanism of this theory is not known, but it is believed that serotonin is part of the response. Our intestines have more serotonin receptors than our brains. Microorganisms in our intestines produce serotonin, which is why these tiny microbes can have a decisive influence on our mental health (Yano et al. 2015, Leclercq et al. 2016).

Melatonin Relieves Bowel Sensitivity

Melatonin may help to strengthen our intestinal health by regulating intestinal mobility, as well as the sensitivity of the gastrointestinal tract to acids. Various studies have shown that melatonin has beneficial effects on irritable bowel syndrome by, among other things, reducing abdominal and rectal pain and improving the associated sleep disturbances. The anti-oxidative effect of melatonin also seems to play a role here (Vaughn et al. 2014).

Circadian Rhythm Affects Gastrointestinal Tract

New research has also shown that melatonin may play an important role in the health of intestinal microbes and their circadian rhythm. As we have already seen, intestinal bacteria also have their own circadian rhythm, which, in turn, influences the functionality of our body and contributes to our health.

An increasing number of studies suggests that these microbes are extremely important to human health, and any imbalance that may be caused by these microbes can result in a disturbance. It is precisely this rhythm of the intestinal bacteria that seems to be synchronized with the circadian processes in our body through melatonin, whether it is produced by the body itself or externally (Vaughn et al. 2014, Bishehsari et al. 2016).

Inflammatory Indications

Inflammatory diseases are on the rise, and the number of diseases increases annually. The most common types are ulcerative colitis (chronic inflammation of the large intestine) and Crohn's disease. Both are recurring episodes of disease, which can occur at a young age, but often in the elderly. If the colitis ulcer affects primarily the intestinal tract and is inflamed, inflammation of the entire digestive tract is seen in Crohn's disease.

Typical Symptoms

Severe abdominal cramps with (usually chronic) diarrhea, abdominal pain, and flatulence are typical symptoms of both diseases. Increased temperature, nausea, and vomiting can also be observed. In the worst cases, fistulae, joint pain, or inflammation of the eyes occurs. The symptoms occur in a pulsatile manner, and the affected people often experience long periods free of any symptoms until a painful, inflammatory phase begins again.

Causes

The causes of inflammatory diseases are not yet clear, but it is assumed that genetic factors can play a role in the development, as do lifestyle choices. A weakened immune system that is no longer able to ward off viruses and bacteria can also lead to the initiation of these inflammatory processes. Stress and depression are also repeatedly connected with these diseases.

Positive Effect of Melatonin

Various studies have shown that melatonin is an important regulator of both inflammation and motility in the gastrointestinal tract, suggesting that complementary melatonin might have a positive effect on large intestinal inflammation (Vaughn et al. 2014). One study even suggests that melatonin can prevent the development of inflammatory diseases (Castanon-Cervantes et al. 2010). (See tables 1 and 2.)

Table 1: Potential impact of the circadian rhythm and sleep on the digestive functions (modified according to Vaughn et al. 2014).		
Digestive function	Impacted by general circadian rhythms	Impacted by sleep-wake rhythm
Saliva production	+/-	+
Swallowing	-	+
Gastric acid production	+	?
Gastric peristaltic	?	+
Nutrient resorption	+	?
Small intestinal peristaltic	+/-	+
Large intestinal peristaltic	+/-	+
Anal function	+/-	+
(=/- = possible; ? = unclear; + = definite impact; -= no impact		

Table 2: Effect mechanisms of melatonin in gastrointestinal diseases (modified according to Vaughn et al. 2014).

Melatonin in the gastrointestinal tract	Cellular effect mechanisms	Clinical presentation of gastrointestinal diseases under melatonin deficiency	First described by
Improvement of the protective mucus production via positive regulation of the circadian rhythm in this organ	Normalization of the endocrine function of the stomach—and duodenum mucosa; reduction of stomach acid production; an increase of the stomach/intestinal blood supply	Stomach and intestinal ulcers	Brzozowski et al. 2007
Optimization of the regeneration of the intestinal mucosa	Normalization of the length of the intestinal villi; optimization of the mucosal regeneration as well as normalization of cell division of the mucosal cells	Intestinal ulcers	Ozturk et al. 2006
Regulation of the circadian rhythm of the intestinal function	Unclear, possibly via the regulation of endogenous zeitgeber in the intestine	Irritable bowel	Enck et al. 2009, Radwan et al. 2009
Multiple anticarcinogenic effects	Unclear, possibly via direct effects on cell division; activation of the programmed cell death; antioxidative effects	Gastrointestinal cancers	Farriol et al. 2000, Anisimov et al. 1997, Anisimov et al. 1999

Inhibition of the formation or reduction of progression of inflammatory intestinal diseases	Unclear, possibly via the synchronization of circadian intestinal rhythm; modification of intestinal permeability; antioxidative effects; improvements of blood supply; immunological effects; improved regeneration	Inflammatory intestinal diseases	Tang et al. 2009
Control of the normal intestinal peristaltic as well as the muscle cell contraction	Optimization of the local serotonin production	Irritable bowel syndrome and/or intestinal cramps	Lange et al. 2010
Reduction of medication-induced colitis	Unclear, possibly via antioxidative effects	Colitis	Castanon-Cervantes et al. 2010

Diabetes

Diabetes mellitus is a widespread metabolic disease that is now considered to be a national disease. In 2012, the disease caused 1.5 million deaths globally. According to estimates published by the WHO in the press release on the Diabetes World Health Day 2016, about 60 million people suffer from diabetes mellitus (WHO 2016).

While older people were affected in the past, more and more young people are now suffering from diabetes. The reason for this lies in our lifestyle, with unhealthy diets and too little exercise. We are becoming increasingly overweight.

In addition, diabetes—both types 1 and 2—are often inherited by future generations. The probability of getting type 2 diabetes if another family member has it is about 50 percent! Common to both types are the increased blood glucose levels (hyperglycemia) caused by a deficiency of insulin.

The consequences of that disease can have dramatic effects, ranging from hypertension, high cholesterol, infectious diseases, strokes, and eye diseases—which in the worst case can lead to blindness, circulatory disorders, and severe inflammation.

Insulin in a Healthy Body

In a healthy body, insulin helps to absorb glucose (a form of sugar we absorb from food) into our blood, which is transported to all the cells of our organs to be consumed. The blood circulation fulfills important functions: our blood contains substances and cells that neutralize pathogens, transports messengers and hormones, and ensures that toxic wastes are transported out of our body. As you can see, our blood plays a vital role in our body and the proper functioning of the whole organism. When sugar reaches target cells via the blood, insulin helps these cells absorb the sugar.

Too Little Insulin Causes Chaos

If the body does not produce enough insulin, however, sugar molecules reach the cells via the blood, but they cannot be absorbed. Instead, sugar floats freely in the blood. The body defends itself against this chaos with all its strength, bringing more and more sugar into the bloodstream, but all in vain. As a consequence, most of the cells of the organs remain unaffected, with the most important nutrients being transported by the glucose. The possible outcome: the already-mentioned disease symptoms.

Insulin Deficiency: Types 1 and 2 Diabetes

Scientists are still researching the exact causes of diabetes. So far, two types are distinguished: type 1 diabetes is an autoimmune disease that mainly affects people starting when they're young. The pancreas, or more precisely, the occurring beta cells, can no longer produce enough insulin; it leads to increased blood glucose levels.

In type 2, the body can no longer release enough insulin, but in this case, it is a metabolic disorder. Type 2 diabetes has a gradual onset, often caused by excess weight and inappropriate dietary habits. The body slowly develops insulin resistance, until hyperglycemia (elevated blood sugar) occurs. Type 2 has long been known as "age diabetes," but adolescents and young adults are increasingly becoming ill as a result of fatty food, lack of exercise, and excess weight.

Influence Factor Lifestyle

It cannot be emphasized enough that lifestyle plays an important role in the development of type 2 diabetes, according to a recent study. We stay awake for too long; are distracted by mobile phones, TV, computers, and permanent light sources; and eat unhealthy diets with too little fruit, vegetables, and vitamins—all of these factors contribute to our sleep-wake rhythm being mixed up. The consequence is that our circadian rhythm—the internal clock—is disturbed, which, in turn, can lead to the metabolic syndrome and thus to diabetes (especially type 2) and fatigue (Sharma et al. 2015).

Numerous studies deal with the influence of sleep and melatonin on the development of diabetes (see, for example, Arora and Taheri 2015) and underline the fact that in addition to genetic factors, lifestyle plays a key role. Scientists have found that a sleep deficit of just half an hour per day can favor diabetes (Arora and Taheri 2015)!

The good news is that another researcher found that the effects of sleep deficit during the week could be compensated by sufficient sleep during the weekend (Broussard et al. 2016).

Correlation between Diabetes and Melatonin Deficiency

All these studies suggest that there is a relationship between low melatonin levels and the development of diabetes. In fact, studies with diabetics have found that their melatonin levels were low. A correlation between sleep disorders and glucose intolerance has also been investigated, which can lead to type 2 diabetes.

Researchers conclude that the circadian rhythm influences hyperglycemia and insulin resistance. The loss of each glycemic control and the increase in glucose in the blood are typical complications that occur in type 2 diabetes and are usually caused by an insulin deficiency, often caused by a lack of function of the beta cells.

Melatonin can improve the function of beta cells and support the release of insulin throughout the day. Melatonin supplementation can thus be a hopeful therapy for those affected (Sharma et al. 2015).

In the Focus: Beta Cells

Beta cells appear to play an essential role in the development of diabetes. Recently, a study that has been published shows that dysfunction and loss of beta cells are potentially responsible for the disease in both types of diabetes. This is a surprising result, as it had been assumed that only type 1 diabetes will destroy the beta cells, and the blood glucose level will subsequently be out of control. The researchers also found that mutations in two genes, XRCC4 and GLIS3, are responsible for the death of the beta cells. The study recommended that drugs be designed to maintain the inherently resistant beta cells instead of replacing their function, as before (Dooley et al. 2016).

Are you wondering what this has to do with melatonin? Remember that melatonin has the ability to regulate the release of insulin and can thus protect cells from overload.

Study Shows Genetic Causes of Diabetes

Scientists assume that gene mutations in the melatonin receptor MTL2 interfere with the link between the internal clock and the release of insulin. This could lead to abnormal blood glucose—and finally to diabetes. Approximately one-third of humanity has a slightly different version of this melatonin receptor in the pancreas, where the beta cells shed insulin. When melatonin binds to the receptors of these cells, secretion slows down. In a mutation, the beta cells react to melatonin by increasing the number of receptors. This enhances the effect that melatonin has on these cells, causing hyperglycemia and other conditions associated with diabetes (Tuomi et al. 2016).

When people who have this genetic variation are working and eating at night while their melatonin levels are high, they have higher blood glucose levels, leading to a greater risk of developing diabetes and other endocrine disorders.

Melatonin Protects against Hyperglycemia

Various studies have shown that melatonin may affect the release of insulin and the blood glucose level (Owino et al. 2016). In rats that were diagnosed with type 2 diabetes, melatonin provided protection from hyperlipidemia (an increase in cholesterol) and hyperglycemia. In mice, there was an improvement in insulin resistance and glucose metabolism. In another study with postmenopausal women, it was found that melatonin improves glucose tolerance and insulin sensitivity in older women.

A further study found that melatonin as an effective antioxidant also improves the efficacy of oral antidiabetics. Considering the fact that melatonin deficiency is especially severe in the elderly, it becomes clear why this particular group of people has an increased risk of diabetes, because melatonin can no longer control the nightly insulin distribution. It is known from animal experiments that melatonin can specifically suppress insulin release via specific receptors. If the nocturnal melatonin is missing, the beta cells release insulin at night, a time when it is not needed (Peschke et al. 2015). It is currently postulated that this increased nighttime release of insulin contributes to the fact that insulin receptors can no longer be formed in the long term, or the insulin receptor can no longer function properly on the body cells. As a result, excess blood sugar and then diabetes develop.

Therapeutic Approach

In the case of people with an increased risk of diabetes, care should be taken to maintain the natural melatonin level, or to maintain it at the correspondingly high level by the additional administration of melatonin. The earlier this hormone replacement therapy begins, the later—if at all—a diabetes disease can occur.

Fertility and Pregnancy

Healthy oocyte production is the first step toward successful conception and a healthy pregnancy. Scientists and doctors have known for years that a healthy sleep rhythm is also important for a healthy menstrual cycle. The perfect interplay of rhythms and cycles in our body is decisively involved in female fertility. If these cycles and rhythms are no longer regular, this can have an influence on the fertility and the course of a pregnancy or the development of the unborn child.

Biological Rhythms and Reproduction

If you are a woman, you may have already experienced your cycle shifting after a long vacation overseas or if after too much stress. Perhaps your menstruation has also been later than usual after unusually challenging, long-lasting physical activity.

Researchers know any disturbance of our circadian rhythm can also shift the menstrual cycle and thus affect fertility (see, e.g., Boden et al. 2013, Reiter et al. 2014c, Reiter et al. 2014d).

Conversely, sleep disturbances, as well as mood fluctuations caused by PMS—premenstrual syndrome—are also factors. Studies with women suffering from PMS have shown that their melatonin level decreases one to two weeks before menstruation, which can be a factor causing these symptoms. Early studies show that chronotherapeutic melatonin and light therapy could help those affected to regulate their melatonin levels, and thus alleviate the symptoms (Shechter and Boivin 2010).

Circadian Disorders Affect Fertility

Jet lag and other circadian rhythmic disorders can have a negative impact on the fertility of a woman, according to many studies that have examined the cycle and the fertility of nurses or flight attendants, for example. It is assumed that the interruption of melatonin production is the root of the problem (Toffol et al. 2016). Female shift workers suffer significantly more from a shift in their cycle than those who do not perform shift work (Baker and Driver 2007).

The Hypothalamic-Pituitary-Ovarian Axis

A complex system controls the fertility of the woman, known as the hypothalamic-pituitary-ovarian axis. The concept of this axis is simple. The hypothalamus sends signals to the pituitary through a hormone called GnRH (gonadotropin releasing hormone). In turn, this stimulates the luteinizing hormone (LH) and the follicle-stimulating hormone (FSH), which trigger the ovaries to produce progesterone and estrogen. These two hormones stimulate a variety of physiological effects, including ovulation, and ultimately control the fertility of women.

The proper functioning of this axis is an excellent example of the close connection and the circadian interplay of these signals, which determine the female cycle. All the mechanisms run after a certain clock stimulated from the outside via the change of light and dark (Toffol et al. 2016).

Melatonin Production in the Female Body

It is proven that melatonin is present in high concentration in the eggs, ovaries, cells around the oocytes, and the placenta. It supports the female reproductive system and protects every cell as an antioxidant from free radicals—especially during ovulation and fertilization (Reiter et al. 2014c).

Researchers have found that the melatonin level increases during pregnancy and reaches its maximum shortly before birth (Voiculescu et al. 2014).

Melatonin Affects the Quality of the Egg Cells

Good egg cells develop embryos that develop just as well. Conversely, this also means poor egg quality is the most common cause of infertility (Tamura et al. 2012). One reason for this is that, like all cells in our body, oocytes are exposed to free radicals. If the defensive mechanism of the female body is not able to ward off these radicals, for example, because of a lack of melatonin, this can have serious consequences for women who wish to get pregnant.

As you have often heard, melatonin is the perfect antioxidant to keep free radicals in check—exemplified by a study by the University of Texas. Melatonin also acts as an antioxidant

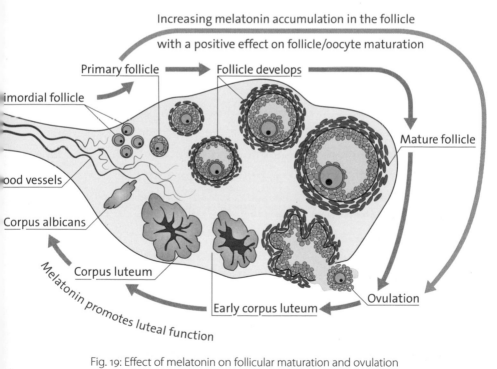

Fig. 19: Effect of melatonin on follicular maturation and ovulation (modified by Reiter et al. 2014b).

in the ovaries by deflecting free radicals and preventing cell damage. In other words, melatonin can also help with infertility. A melatonin treatment during the period when a woman wants to get pregnant shows improved prospects, as the chance of fertilization and the rate of pregnancy are considerably increased (Reiter et al. 2014b). (See Fig. 19.)

Recently, a study found that melatonin promotes the maturation of oocytes and mitochondria, which assume important functions of energy production in the cell. Surprisingly, the scientists found that mitochondria are also the most important production sites for the melatonin synthesis in oocytes and that, in turn, melatonin improves the function of these mitochondria and ultimately protects the cells from free radicals. The researchers concluded that melatonin improves the quality of the eggs and accelerates the development capacity of embryos, not just after in vitro fertilization (IVF) treatment (He et al. 2016).

Melatonin Supports Success of In Vitro Fertilization

Researchers have found that women who undergo IVF treatment and who take melatonin have greater chances of becoming pregnant and giving birth to a healthy child. For this purpose, women with a very low fertility rate were given 3 mg of melatonin for one month before undergoing IVF treatment again. The amazing results concluded that melatonin input increased the gestation rate by 50 percent (Tamura et al. 2008, Tamura et al. 2009)!

Melatonin Supports Fetal Development

Another chronobiological study found that melatonin is essential for embryonic and fetal development of the unborn child. Why is that? The melatonin level of the expectant mother increases constantly during pregnancy and supplies the unborn child directly via the placenta. This maternal melatonin, which can also be detected in the amniotic fluid, has various functions for the fetus. On the one hand, it conveys information about light and dark cycles to the brain of the unborn child, which helps the child to form his own circadian rhythm. Although the fetal brain already has its own melatonin receptors, they have not yet fully developed and can be influenced by melatonin. On the other hand, it is assumed that melatonin also plays an important role in the activation of certain genes that are important from conception to birth. Melatonin promotes the development of the fetal SCN and can lead to subsequent behavioral problems of the child in the case of melatonin deficiency (Reiter et al. 2014b).

Therefore, various scientists recommend melatonin supplementation for pregnant women, especially when sleeping problems occur. For the unborn child, the effects of melatonin are only positive; no negative effects have been demonstrated (Voiculescu et al. 2014).

Melatonin Promotes Embryonic Development

Melatonin is an important regulator of the fetal development process:

> It supports the circadian rhythm in the unborn child.
> It seems to have a direct influence on the development of the nervous and endocrine systems.
> It protects the organs responsible for the metabolism of the unborn child from oxidative stress.
> It reduces the risk of long-term health disparities due to complicated pregnancies (Voiculescu et al. 2014).

Study: Dysfunction of the Placenta due to Melatonin Deficiency

The placenta plays a very important role in pregnancy; it is the child's care center. Communication and exchanges between the mother and the child are carried out by means of this tissue to which the child is connected by the umbilical cord (see Fig. 20).

If there are complications during pregnancy, it is usually due to a problem with the placenta. If its function is disturbed, this can lead to dramatic consequences for mother and child, such as spontaneous abortion, premature birth, premature placental solution, or preeclampsia (Valenzuela et al. 2015).

Preeclampsia is a disorder that occurs during pregnancy in which the woman has very high blood pressure. Also, the protein content in the urine is increased in women with this disease. To date, this has been associated with a dysfunction of the placenta and oxidative stress. A recently published study showed that melatonin deficiency could also be a risk factor for placental dysfunction during pregnancy (Zeng et al. 2016).

Older studies show that women with preeclampsia have markedly reduced melatonin levels (Nakamura et al. 2001); the placenta of these women also showed low melatonin levels (Lanoix et al. 2012). With its antioxidant effect, melatonin can protect the placenta from free radicals that are toxic in preeclampsia and regulate the blood pressure of pregnant women.

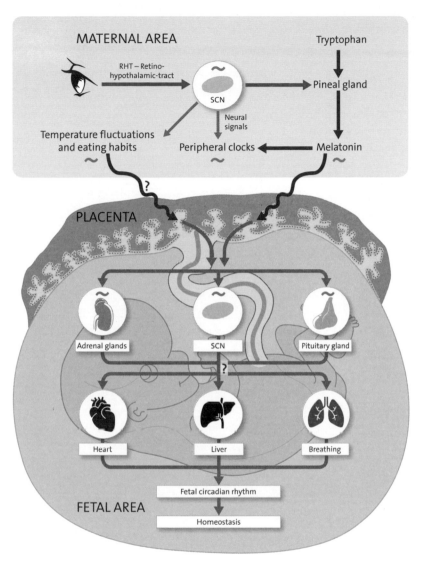

Fig. 20: Complex linkage of maternal circadian melatonin secretion or maternal biorhythms with the development of the rhythmicity of the unborn child (modified according to Reiter et al., 2014c).

Pregnancy in Diabetics

Children of diabetics have an increased risk of developing a metabolic disorder during adulthood. Also, a connection with a later cardiovascular disease is always suspected. A study has confirmed this assumption in animal experiments and has shown that melatonin, when administered during pregnancy, can significantly reduce the risk of subsequent heart disease in the child (Gao et al. 2016).

Fertility? Ensure a Healthy Melatonin Level

Optimal fertility requires a healthy melatonin level. Many studies show that if the expectant mother is exposed to light during pregnancy, this has an impact on the development of the embryo.

Researchers recommend that pregnant women maintain a regular sleep-wake rhythm, especially in the last trimester of pregnancy, to maintain their natural melatonin at a healthy level. Long-flight trips, especially over several time zones, are discouraged, as well as long-term stays in artificial light. Be aware that all of this affects your circadian rhythm and harms your child (Reiter et al. 2014b).

Cancer

While melatonin has been used for decades for the treatment of insomnia and other sleep disorders, it could also be extremely valuable in the treatment of cancer, because for cancers, the right timing is crucial in many respects. Normal cells grow and die due to very rhythmic processes, which are defined by so-called watch genes. When these genes mutate or otherwise function abnormally, cells can grow uncontrolled and kill healthy cells in their vicinity.

Melatonin in the Fight against Cancer

Studies on melatonin as an anticancer hormone have existed for fifty years. All these studies show that the receptor MTL1 is mainly involved. Melatonin has a direct influence on tumor growth and, in parallel, has an antioxidant effect. Scientists recommend that melatonin, due to its nontoxic properties, low costs, and easy and fast availability, should be taken into consideration in clinical treatment (Hill et al. 2015).

Risk Factor: Disturbed Day-Night Rhythm

Recent studies suggest that melatonin inhibits the growth of the tumor, while alleviating the negative side effects of some cancer therapies. It has been shown several times that people who work at night instead of sleeping show a higher risk of cancer, which is why the WHO classified shift work as a carcinogen (i.e., a cancer-promoting factor). Studies repeatedly establish a connection between night shift work and cancer (Benabu et al. 2015).

Although the link between an interrupted circadian rhythm and cancer is unambiguous, the mechanism of the increased risk of cancer has so far been unknown.

Slowed Tumor Growth

A new analysis of chronobiology studies suggests that melatonin interferes with cancer at its foundation by breaking the biochemical processes that cause tumors to grow (Vinther and Claësson 2015). When laboratory animals suffering from tumors were supplied with melatonin, tumor growth slowed considerably. In addition, studies show that human cancer patients can better tolerate other treatments when they take melatonin. In the near future, the "miracle hormone" could become a fixed part of the standard cancer treatment, according to the unanimous opinion of experts.

Melatonin in the Treatment of Cancer

For years, science has devoted itself to the effects of melatonin on a variety of cancers (Rondanelli et al. 2013). The common conviction is that melatonin is an "intelligent killer" of cancer cells. It protects the healthy cells from attacks and triggers self-destruction in cancer cells (Bizzarri et al. 2013).

Melatonin in Chemotherapy and Radiation Therapy

For a long time, science has been concerned with melatonin and its positive effect with chemo- and radiotherapy. Melatonin has long proved itself to help with its toxic side effects; at the same time, it acts as an antioxidant and thus promotes the programmed death of cancer cells.

A study investigated tumor patients who were suffering from lung, breast, stomach, brain, and neck cancer. One group was treated with melatonin in parallel to the chemotherapy, and the other group was treated exclusively with chemotherapy. The result was that a one-year survival rate and tumor decline were significantly higher in patients treated with melatonin as opposed to those who received chemotherapy alone (Lissoni et al. 1999).

A few years later, a similar study with tumor patients came to the same conclusion. The decline in the tumor and the two-year survival rate were significantly higher in those patients who were also treated with melatonin in parallel to chemotherapy. These studies clearly show that melatonin can increase the efficacy of any cancer treatment (Lissoni 2007).

If applied in a preventive fashion, melatonin could also reduce the long-term cancer risk of X-rays, according to a recent study. The first animal tests are very promising, and there is hope that the great potential of melatonin will also be applied here (Zetner et al. 2016).

"Natural Killer" Melatonin

As a natural killer, melatonin plays an important role in the function of cells: it inhibits the uncontrolled proliferation of cells, thus reducing tumor growth, and can even prevent tumor formation by activating the lymphocytes (Zamfir Chiru et al. 2014). Melatonin also protects against common toxic consequences of chemotherapy or radiation, such as nausea and vomiting, low blood pressure, and lack of strength by stimulating the immune system (Seely et al. 2012). Melatonin also relieves inflammation of the oral mucosa, reduces harmful effects on the heart, and helps to reduce blood glucose and insufficient numbers of blood platelets after chemotherapy (Lissoni 2002).

Warburg Effect in Cancer

Studies also show that melatonin not only inhibits tumor growth and the proliferation of cancer cells, but also suppresses the so-called Warburg effect (Mao et al. 2016). This is a theory of physician and biochemist Otto Warburg, who observed that glucose metabolism plays a major role in the growth of tumor cells. If glucose is broken down in the body, lactate is formed. In a healthy person, it enters the mitochondria, where it provides energy. Unfortunately, this energy generation also produces free radicals that kill cells. In tumor cells, the mitochondria do not absorb the lactate, which means that they produce less energy but also no free radicals. The reduced energy production is then compensated by an increased sugar consumption of these cells, according to Warburg's assumption.

Scientists have shown that a suppressed melatonin release at night, due to nocturnal light sources, can favor the Warburg effect and thus the development and growth of tumors. On the other hand, an evening dose of melatonin suppressed the Warburg effect (Blask et al. 2014).

Breast Cancer

Scientists have long been convinced that the disturbance of the day-night rhythm can have an impact on the development of breast cancer (Pillittere and Miller 2000, Leonardi et al. 2012). A study with women who have been working in shifts for more than twenty years and suffering from sleep disorders came to the conclusion that they are more likely to develop breast cancer than women in occupations with regulated working hours and normal sleep (Benabu et al. 2015).

Sleep and Light Quality Affect Breast Cancer

Scientists are continually investigating whether and how much nightly light increases the risk of developing breast cancer—with astonishing results. For example, a study of women's sleep and lighting habits were evaluated, including their sleep quality, bedtimes, falling asleep with either more television or reading, and the type and intensity of the lighting. The women who slept longer and in the darkened room read a book before sleeping with a special reading lamp developed breast cancer less frequently (Keshet-Sitton et al. 2016).

The influence of light and physical activity on melatonin production was investigated by an older study and concluded that regular, even moderate movement during the day positively influences the melatonin level and thus has a protective influence on breast cancer risk (Knight et al. 2005).

The doctors therefore recommend a sleeping period of six to eight hours, which can prevent breast cancer. If you are a woman, you should take this recommendation to heart!

Melatonin in Breast Cancer

Melatonin plays an important role in the fight against cancer, not only as a potent antioxidant. Many studies have shown that melatonin has a direct influence on various malignant tumors. It can affect tumor growth in some types of breast cancer by directly reducing the cell division rate. In addition, it also affects the activity of estrogens on these cells, which play an important role in breast cancer. Melatonin also reduces the aggressiveness of the tumor and the side effects of radiotherapy and chemotherapy (Sánchez-Barceló et al. 2012).

Recently, scientists have shown that melatonin can also prevent cell migration and invasion. This protects our body from the spread of lethal tumor cells into new tissue (Gonçalves et al. 2016b).

Melatonin can also positively influence the tumor weight and thus tumor size, a prerequisite required by many therapists before any chemotherapy or surgery is performed (Ma et al. 2015).

Melatonin Inhibits Tumor Growth

Recently, a study showed that melatonin not only inhibits the growth of breast cancer cells, but also the new formation and growth of blood vessels (angiogenesis). This is an important finding, because these vessels provide the tumor with oxygen and nutrients and thus contribute to its growth.

Melatonin also reduces uncontrolled cell division, the so-called telomerase activity, and the uncontrolled spread of cancer cells into other tissues. Increased telomerase activity allows the tumor cell to constantly divide and penetrate into other tissues. Melatonin is one of the few substances that can reduce this activity, especially in tumor cells, thus reducing the formation of metastases. What is also underlined in the study is that melatonin supports programmed cell death or apoptosis, alleviates the serious side effects of chemotherapeutic agents, and simultaneously increases the efficacy of chemotherapy and radiation therapy. The authors of the study conclude that its broad spectrum of effects makes melatonin a treatment agent that can achieve very positive effects in breast cancer treatment (Nooshinfar et al. 2017).

Radiotherapy and the Healing Process

As a pretreatment of chemotherapy or radiotherapy, melatonin can significantly sensitize breast cancer cells, according to a recent study. Melatonin reduces the activity and expression of certain proteins by about 50 percent, thereby reducing the amount of bioactive estrogens that promote tumor growth (Alonso-González et al. 2016). Melatonin also demonstrated excellent efficacy after breast cancer surgeries and improved patient sleep quality—an important effect for the regeneration phase and the healing process of women (Madsen et al. 2016b).

Colon Cancer

In colorectal cancer, good results can be reported with a parallel melatonin input. In one study, colorectal cancer patients were treated with chemotherapy combined with daily melatonin. Despite low doses, chemotherapy showed a higher efficacy due to melatonin (Cerea et al. 2003).

A recent clinical study investigated the influence of melatonin on chemotherapy in other colon cancer patients. The scientists concluded that melatonin significantly increases the chemotherapeutic effect of 5-fluorouracil, which is usually used in colorectal cancer (Gao et al. 2016).

Skin Cancer

Sunlight is important for our mood, our body, and our health. Nevertheless, it can become a risk factor. UV radiation is one of the main causes of skin cancer—and it's on the rise. We are permanently generating free radicals, which can attack our body. Melatonin as the perfect body-borne antioxidant can become a key figure in the fight against skin cancer, as is confirmed time and time again in many studies (Goswami and Haldar 2015). Melatonin receptors, found in our skin and their cells, fulfill important functions such as cell regeneration. In addition, melatonin provides good protection against free radicals by UV radiation (Slominski et al. 2014).

Melatonin Protects against Melanoma

Scientists have long been concerned with the relationship between circadian rhythm and skin cancer, especially melanoma. Studies with firefighters, flight attendants, pilots, and nurses confirm that melanomas are increasingly found in people who do shift work (Gutierrez and Arbesman 2016). A disturbed day-night rhythm has a negative effect on the repair mechanisms, which follow a circadian rhythm and depend on melatonin signals.

Many studies show that melatonin can help protect against the serious effects of UV radiation, but only if it is applied as a cream before sunbathing. However, it does not have any effect when it is used only afterward (Scheuer et al. 2014).

Lung Cancer

In the case of lung cancer, studies show a correlation with a disturbed day-night rhythm. For example, researchers have demonstrated that jet lag can promote the development and progression of lung tumors. It is mainly two genes that play a tumor-suppressing role in the cells. However, they cannot fulfill this important function if the circadian rhythm is disturbed. Uncontrolled cell growth is the result—a fatal situation for the healthy cells that can no longer fight against the tumor cells (Papagiannakopoulos et al. 2016). A direct effect of melatonin on these genes has not yet been demonstrated but is accepted by many scientists. The first clinical studies on melatonin in lung cancer therapy suggest a therapeutic benefit (Habtemariam et al. 2017).

Stomach Cancer

Similar results have also been achieved in patients with gastric cancer, where melatonin shows its great anticancer effect. It inhibits the spread of lethal tumor cells, and thus of metastases, and promotes programmed cell death (Zhang et al. 2013).

In an experiment in which tumor cells were treated with melatonin, the behavior of the malignant cells was directly affected. It not only inhibited the viability of the cells, but also hindered cloning and spreading into healthy tissue. Again, the researchers strongly recommend that melatonin be considered as an effective antitumor agent or supporting therapy (Li et al. 2015).

Prostate Cancer

Prostate cancer affects more than 13 percent of men and is thus considered a very common cancer. Like breast cancer, prostate cancer appears to be associated with too little sleep. A study concluded that this was mainly true for men who had late stage prostate cancer. Further, the investigation found that men who work in long and irregular shifts are more likely to develop prostate cancer (Gapstur et al. 2014).

The relationship between circadian rhythm and prostate cancer is emphasized in a recently published study and underlines the extremely positive effects of melatonin parallel to radiotherapy or chemotherapy, both in terms of increased efficacy and reduced toxicity (Kiss and Ghosh 2016).

Animal Experiments with Melatonin

The fluid of the prostate gland serves the transport of sperm and contains very high concentrations of glucose. An animal experiment found that melatonin inhibits the growth of the tumor, which is favored by the high glucose content of the glandular fluid, which is reminiscent of the Warburg effect, thus prolonging the mice's lives (Hevia et al. 2015).

In a further animal experiment, melatonin increased the survival of mice with prostate cancer by 33 percent—regardless of whether the melatonin was administered at the beginning or during the advanced stage of the tumor (Mayo et al. 2017). If these effects are confirmed in humans, this would be another indication for melatonin in practice.

Summary and Outlook

Melatonin research over recent decades—from the first mention of the pineal gland to the time of the discovery of the hormone produced by this gland, to this day—has revealed new knowledge for our health. Admittedly, not all the theses have turned out to be correct. Just think of the historical retrospect at the beginning of this book, where the seat of the soul and movement were concerned. But what could be confirmed is that melatonin and its effects in our bodies are of great importance for our health.

"Sleep well" is age-old wisdom—even today, research is being conducted on how healthy sleep affects our bodies. Melatonin is always the focus, as the scientific evidence suggests that a natural release of melatonin is a basic prerequisite for achieving an old age in full health, without major diseases, if possible. In recent decades, the responsible mechanisms have been partially deciphered and thus show new therapeutic approaches to better treat sleep disorders, a still-underestimated national disease. The goal of the next few years must be to raise awareness of this often-trivialized disease and to treat people with sleep disorders with appropriate measures.

Since the discovery that melatonin is a perfect antioxidant, that is to say it neutralizes free radicals, interest in this field has increased and continues to do so today. The great utility of melatonin in many diseases caused by inflammation has already been demonstrated, but researchers are working to decipher further possibilities. Experience shows that the targeted use of melatonin, even if only as supplemental medication, can be of immense help not only in tumor control, but also in myocardial infarction and stroke. If these effects can be confirmed by further studies in the future, we can assume that melatonin will be used as a standard therapy in these diseases in a few years. Melatonin also has an antioxidant effect when it comes to reducing the side effects of some drugs or increasing their efficacy. Here, too, a new field of research opens up, and the benefits an additional dose of melatonin will have on these established therapies can be eagerly awaited.

A still relatively young research area in which melatonin plays a key role is chronobiology. Recognizing that daily fluctuations of various body functions are of great importance helped establish chronobiology and the associated areas, such as chronophysiology, chronopharmacology, and chronotherapy, as research areas. It is already known that changes in the circadian release of melatonin often have negative effects on our health. Encouraging first results of investigations of how melatonin and light therapy can reconcile disturbances between external timers, such as light and darkness, and internal clocks such as melatonin are now available. Disorders of this equilibrium, or chronodisruption, in the future will increasingly become the focus of science in order to better understand the connections between internal clocks and the development of tumors, diabetes, hypertension, and other human diseases. Further fields for the therapeutic use of melatonin as a universal timer will be opened. Studies that analyze the effect of melatonin on specific cell structures or certain genes already suggest promising new fields of application.

Let us sum up: "*Mens sana in corpore sano,*" meaning "a healthy mind in a healthy body," is something the ancient Romans had already recognized. Today, we know that sufficient sleep or sufficient melatonin is of great importance for health. Thus, the Greek philosophers might perhaps have been right when they gave the pineal gland, with melatonin as its messenger, immense importance. The seat of the soul will presumably never be exactly determined, but melatonin is different. We can assume that science will provide us with new insights into the subject that we cannot yet imagine. Thus, the last chapter on the topic of melatonin and the secrets of this wonderful hormone is certainly not yet written.

List of Sources

Abbott, Sabra M., and Phyllis C. Zee. 2015. "Irregular Sleep-Wake Rhythm Disorder." *Sleep Medicine Clinics* 10 (4): 517–22. https://doi.org/10.1016/j.jsmc.2015.08.005.

Alagiakrishnan, Kannayiram. 2016. "Melatonin Based Therapies for Delirium and Dementia." *Discovery Medicine* 21 (117): 363–71.

Allagui, Mohamed S., Rafik Hachani, Saber Saidi, Anouer Feriani, Jean C. Murat, Kamel Kacem, and Abdelfatteh El feki. 2015. "Pleiotropic Protective Roles of Melatonin against Aluminium-Induced Toxicity in Rats." *General Physiology and Biophysics* 34 (4): 415–24. https://doi.org/10.4149/gpb_2015028.

Almeida, Eduardo Alves de, Paolo Di Mascio, Tatsuo Harumi, D. Warren Spence, Adam Moscovitch, Rüdiger Hardeland, Daniel P. Cardinali, Gregory M. Brown, and S. R. Pandi-Perumal. 2011. "Measurement of Melatonin in Body Fluids: Standards, Protocols and Procedures." *Child's Nervous System: ChNS: Official Journal of the International Society for Pediatric Neurosurgery* 27 (6): 879–91. https://doi.org/10.1007/s00381-010-1278-8.

Alonso-González, Carolina, Alicia González, Carlos Martínez-Campa, Javier Menéndez-Menéndez, José Gómez-Arozamena, Angela García-Vidal, and Samuel Cos. 2016. "Melatonin Enhancement of the Radiosensitivity of Human Breast Cancer Cells Is Associated with the Modulation of Proteins Involved in Estrogen Biosynthesis." *Cancer Letters* 370 (1): 145–52. https://doi.org/10.1016/j.canlet.2015.10.015.

Alstadhaug, Karl, Rolf Salvesen, and Svein Bekkelund. 2007. "Insomnia and Circadian Variation of Attacks in Episodic Migraine." *Headache: The Journal of Head and Face Pain* 47 (8): 1184–88. https://doi.org/10.1111/j.1526-4610.2007.00858.x.

Altman, Brian J., Annie L. Hsieh, Arjun Sengupta, Saikumari Y. Krishnanaiah, Zachary E. Stine, Zandra E. Walton, Arvin M. Gouw, et al. 2015. "MYC Disrupts the Circadian Clock and Metabolism in Cancer Cells." *Cell Metabolism* 22 (6): 1009–19. https://doi.org/10.1016/j.cmet.2015.09.003.

Ambriz-Tututi, Mónica, Héctor I. Rocha-González, Silvia L. Cruz, and Vinicio Granados-Soto. 2009. "Melatonin: A Hormone That Modulates Pain." *Life Sciences* 84 (15–16): 489–98. https://doi.org/10.1016/j.lfs.2009.01.024.

Amstrup, Anne Kristine, Tanja Sikjaer, Steen B. Pedersen, Lene Heickendorff, Leif Mosekilde, and Lars Rejnmark. 2016. "Reduced Fat Mass and Increased Lean Mass in Response to 1 Year of Melatonin Treatment in

Postmenopausal Women: A Randomized Placebo-Controlled Trial." *Clinical Endocrinology* 84 (3): 342–47. https://doi.org/10.1111/cen.12942.

Andersen, Lars P. H., Mads U. Werner, Mette M. Rosenkilde, Nathja G. Harpsøe, Hanne Fuglsang, Jacob Rosenberg, and Ismail Gögenur. 2016. "Pharmacokinetics of Oral and Intravenous Melatonin in Healthy Volunteers." *BMC Pharmacology and Toxicology* 17 (1): 8. https://doi.org/10.1186/s40360-016-0052-2.

Andersen, Lars Peter Holst, Ismail Gögenur, Jacob Rosenberg, and Russel J. Reiter. 2016. "Pharmacokinetics of Melatonin: The Missing Link in Clinical Efficacy?" *Clinical Pharmacokinetics* 55 (9): 1027–30. https://doi.org/10.1007/s40262-016-0386-3.

Andrabi, Syed Suhail, Suhel Parvez, and Heena Tabassum. 2015. "Melatonin and Ischemic Stroke: Mechanistic Roles and Action." *Advances in Pharmacological Sciences.* https://doi.org/10.1155/2015/384750.

Anisimov, V. N., I. G. Popovich, and M. A. Zabezhinski. 1997. "Melatonin and Colon Carcinogenesis: I. Inhibitory Effect of Melatonin on Development of Intestinal Tumors Induced by 1,2-Dimethylhydrazine in Rats." *Carcinogenesis* 18 (8): 1549–53. https://doi.org/10.1093/carcin/18.8.1549.

Arbon, Emma L., Malgorzata Knurowska, and Derk-Jan Dijk. 2015. "Randomised Clinical Trial of the Effects of Prolonged-Release Melatonin, Temazepam and Zolpidem on Slow-Wave Activity during Sleep in Healthy People." *Journal of Psychopharmacology* 29 (7): 764–76. https://doi.org/10.1177/0269881115581963.

Arendt, J. 1995. *Melatonin and the Mammalian Pineal Gland.* London: Chapman and Hall.

Arora, Teresa, and Shahrad Taheri. 2015. "Sleep Optimization and Diabetes Control: A Review of the Literature." *Diabetes Therapy* 6 (4): 425–68. https://doi.org/10.1007/s13300-015-0141-z.

Aschoff, Jürgen, and Johannes Meyer-Lohmann. 1955. "Die Aktivitätsperiodik von Nagern im künstlichen 24-Stunden-Tag mit 6–20 Stunden lichtzeit." *Zeitschrift für vergleichende Physiologie* 37 (2): 107–17. https://doi.org/10.1007/BF00298546.

Baandrup, Lone, Birgitte Fagerlund, and Birte Glenthoj. 2017. "Neurocognitive Performance, Subjective Well-Being, and Psychosocial Functioning after Benzodiazepine Withdrawal in Patients with Schizophrenia or Bipolar Disorder: A Randomized Clinical Trial of Add-on Melatonin versus Placebo." *European Archives of Psychiatry and Clinical Neuroscience* 267 (2): 163–71. https://doi.org/10.1007/s00406-016-0711-8.

Baker, Fiona C., and Helen S. Driver. 2007. "Circadian Rhythms, Sleep, and the Menstrual Cycle." *Sleep Medicine*, Circadian Rhythms in Sleep Medicine, 8 (6): 613–22. https://doi.org/10.1016/j.sleep.2006.09.011.

Barloese, Mads Christian Johannes. 2015. "Neurobiology and Sleep Disorders in Cluster Headache." *Journal of Headache and Pain* 16 (1): 78. https://doi.org/10.1186/s10194-015-0562-0.

Beesley, Stephen, Justin Lee, and James Olcese. 2015. "Circadian Clock Regulation of Melatonin MTNR1B Receptor Expression in Human Myometrial Smooth Muscle Cells." *MHR: Basic Science of Reproductive Medicine* 21 (8): 662–71. https://doi.org/10.1093/molehr/gav023.

Belancio, Victoria P. 2015. "LINE-1 Activity as Molecular Basis for Genomic Instability Associated with Light Exposure at Night." *Mobile Genetic Elements* 5 (3): 46–50. https://doi.org/10.1080/2159256X.2015.1037416.

Benabu, J. C., F. Stoll, M. Gonzalez, and C. Mathelin. 2015. "Night Work, Shift Work: Breast Cancer Risk Factor?" *Gynecologie, Obstetrique & Fertilite* 43 (12): 791–99. https://doi.org/10.1016/j.gyobfe.2015.10.004.

Bhatti, Parveen, Dana K. Mirick, Timothy W. Randolph, Jicheng Gong, Diana Taibi Buchanan, Junfeng (Jim) Zhang, and Scott Davis. 2016. "Oxidative DNA Damage during Sleep Periods among Nightshift Workers." *Occupational & Environmental Medicine* 73 (8): 537–44. https://doi.org/10.1136/oemed-2016-103629.

Bishehsari, Faraz, Francis Levi, Fred W. Turek, and Ali Keshavarzian. 2016. "Circadian Rhythms in Gastrointestinal Health and Diseases." *Gastroenterology* 151 (3): e1–5. https://doi.org/10.1053/j.gastro.2016.07.036.

Bizzarri, Mariano, Sara Proietti, Alessandra Cucina, and Russel J. Reiter. 2013. "Molecular Mechanisms of the Pro-Apoptotic Actions of Melatonin in Cancer: A Review." *Expert Opinion on Therapeutic Targets* 17 (12): 1483–96. https://doi.org/10.1517/14728222.2013.834890.

Blasiak, Janusz, Russel J. Reiter, and Kai Kaarniranta. 2016. "Melatonin in Retinal Physiology and Pathology: The Case of Age-Related Macular Degeneration." *Oxidative Medicine and Cellular Longevity*. https://doi.org/10.1155/2016/6819736.

Blask, David E., Robert T. Dauchy, Erin M. Dauchy, Lulu Mao, Steven M. Hill, Michael W. Greene, Victoria P. Belancio, Leonard A. Sauer, and Leslie Davidson. 2014. "Light Exposure at Night Disrupts Host/Cancer Circadian Regulatory Dynamics: Impact on the Warburg Effect, Lipid Signaling and Tumor Growth Prevention." *PLOS ONE* 9 (8): e102776. https://doi.org/10.1371/journal.pone.0102776.

Blum, Ian D., Lei Zhu, Luc Moquin, Maia V. Kokoeva, Alain Gratton, Bruno Giros, and Kai-Florian Storch. 2014. "A Highly Tunable Dopaminergic Oscillator Generates Ultradian Rhythms of Behavioral Arousal." ELife. https://doi.org/10.7554/eLife.05105.

Boden, M. J., T. J. Varcoe, and D. J. Kennaway. 2013. "Circadian Regulation of Reproduction: From Gamete to Offspring." *Progress in Biophysics and*

Molecular Biology 113 (3): 387–97. https://doi.org/10.1016/j
.pbiomolbio.2013.01.003.

Bonmati-Carrion, Maria Angeles, Raquel Arguelles-Prieto, Maria Jose
Martinez-Madrid, Russel Reiter, Ruediger Hardeland, Maria Angeles
Rol, and Juan Antonio Madrid. 2014. "Protecting the Melatonin Rhythm
through Circadian Healthy Light Exposure." *International Journal of
Molecular Sciences* 15 (12): 23448–500. https://doi.org/10.3390
/ijms151223448.

Breen, David P., Cristina Nombela, Romina Vuono, P. Simon Jones, Kate
Fisher, David J. Burn, David J. Brooks, Akhilesh B. Reddy, James B. Rowe,
and Roger A. Barker. 2016. "Hypothalamic Volume Loss Is Associated
with Reduced Melatonin Output in Parkinson's Disease." *Movement
Disorders* 31 (7): 1062–66. https://doi.org/10.1002/mds.26592.

Breus, Michael. 2016. *The Power of When: Discover Your Chronotype—and the
Best Time to Eat Lunch, Ask for a Raise, Have Sex, Write a Novel, Take Your
Meds, and More.* New York: Little, Brown.

Broussard, Josiane L., Kristen Wroblewski, Jennifer M. Kilkus, and Esra
Tasali. 2016. "Two Nights of Recovery Sleep Reverses the Effects of Short-
Term Sleep Restriction on Diabetes Risk." *Diabetes Care* 39 (3): e40–41.
https://doi.org/10.2337/dc15-2214.

Brzozowski, T., K. Zwirska-Korczala, P. C. Konturek, S. J. Konturek, Z.
Sliwowski, M. Pawlik, S. Kwiecien, et al. 2007. "Role of Circadian Rhythm
and Endogenous Melatonin in Pathogenesis of Acute Gastric Bleeding
Erosions Induced by Stress." *Journal of Physiology and Pharmacology: An
Official Journal of the Polish Physiological Society* 58 Suppl 6 (December):
53–64.

Burke, Tina M., Rachel R. Markwald, Andrew W. McHill, Evan D. Chinoy,
Jesse A. Snider, Sara C. Bessman, Christopher M. Jung, John S. O'Neill,
and Kenneth P. Wright. 2015. "Effects of Caffeine on the Human Circadian
Clock in Vivo and in Vitro." *Science Translational Medicine* 7 (305):
305ra146. https://doi.org/10.1126/scitranslmed.aac5125.

Cagnacci, Angelo, Marianna Cannoletta, Antonietta Renzi, Francesco
Baldassari, Serenella Arangino, and Annibale Volpe. 2005. "Prolonged
Melatonin Administration Decreases Nocturnal Blood Pressure in
Women." *American Journal of Hypertension* 18 (12): 1614–18. https://doi
.org/10.1016/j.amjhyper.2005.05.008.

Cagnacci, Angelo, Serenella Arangino, Antonietta Renzi, Anna Maria
Paoletti, Gian Benedetto Melis, Paolo Cagnacci, and Annibale Volpe.
2001. "Influence of Melatonin Administration on Glucose Tolerance and
Insulin Sensitivity of Postmenopausal Women." *Clinical Endocrinology* 54
(3): 339–46. https://doi.org/10.1046/j.1365-2265.2001.01232.x.

Carabotti, Marilia, Annunziata Scirocco, Maria Antonietta Maselli, and Carola Severi. 2015. "The Gut-Brain Axis: Interactions between Enteric Microbiota, Central and Enteric Nervous Systems." *Annals of Gastroenterology: Quarterly Publication of the Hellenic Society of Gastroenterology* 28 (2): 203–9.

Carpenter, Joanne S., Amy C. Abelmann, Sean N. Hatton, Rébecca Robillard, Daniel F. Hermens, Maxwell R. Bennett, Jim Lagopoulos, and Ian B. Hickie. 2017. "Pineal Volume and Evening Melatonin in Young People with Affective Disorders." *Brain Imaging and Behavior* 11 (6): 1741–50. https://doi.org/10.1007/s11682-016-9650-2.

Castanon-Cervantes, Oscar, Mingwei Wu, J. Christopher Ehlen, Ketema Paul, Karen L. Gamble, Russell L. Johnson, Rachel C. Besing, Michael Menaker, Andrew T. Gewirtz, and Alec J. Davidson. 2010. "Dysregulation of Inflammatory Responses by Chronic Circadian Disruption." *Journal of Immunology* 185 (10): 5796–5805. https://doi.org/10.4049/jimmunol.1001026.

Celinski, Krzysztof, P.C. Konturek, M. Slomka, H. Cichoz-Lach, Thomas Brzozowski, S.J. Konturek, and Agnieszka Korolczuk. 2014. "Effects of Treatment with Melatonin and Tryptophan on Liver Enzymes, Parameters of Fat Metabolism and Plasma Levels of Cytokines in Patients with Non-Alcoholic Fatty Liver Disease—14 Months Follow Up." *Journal of Physiology and Pharmacology: An Official Journal of the Polish Physiological Society* 65 (February): 75–82.

Cerea, G., M. Vaghi, A. Ardizzoia, S. Villa, R. Bucovec, S. Mengo, G. Gardani, G. Tancini, and P. Lissoni. 2003. "Biomodulation of Cancer Chemotherapy for Metastatic Colorectal Cancer: A Randomized Study of Weekly Low-Dose Irinotecan Alone versus Irinotecan plus the Oncostatic Pineal Hormone Melatonin in Metastatic Colorectal Cancer Patients Progressing on 5-Fluorouracil-Containing Combinations." *Anticancer Research* 23 (2C): 1951–54.

Chang, Anne-Marie, Andrew C. Bjonnes, Daniel Aeschbach, Orfeu M. Buxton, Joshua J. Gooley, Clare Anderson, Eliza Van Reen, et al. 2016a. "Circadian Gene Variants Influence Sleep and the Sleep Electroencephalogram in Humans." *Chronobiology International* 33 (5): 561–73. https://doi.org/10.3109/07420528.2016.1167078.

Chang, Anne-Marie, Daniel Aeschbach, Jeanne F. Duffy, and Charles A. Czeisler. 2015. "Evening Use of Light-Emitting EReaders Negatively Affects Sleep, Circadian Timing, and next-Morning Alertness." *Proceedings of the National Academy of Sciences of the United States of America* 112 (4): 1232–37. https://doi.org/10.1073/pnas.1418490112.

Chang, Yung-Sen, Ming-Hung Lin, Jyh-Hong Lee, Pei-Lin Lee, Yang-Shia Dai, Kuan-Hua Chu, Chi Sun, et al. 2016b. "Melatonin Supplementation for Children with Atopic Dermatitis and Sleep Disturbance: A Randomized Clinical Trial." *JAMA Pediatrics* 170 (1): 35–42. https://doi.org/10.1001/jamapediatrics.2015.3092.

Chen, Chong, Chong Chen, Caixia Xu, Caixia Xu, Taifeng Zhou, Taifeng Zhou, Bo Gao, et al. 2016a. "Abnormal Osteogenic and Chondrogenic Differentiation of Human Mesenchymal Stem Cells from Patients with Adolescent Idiopathic Scoliosis in Response to Melatonin." *Molecular Medicine Reports* 14 (2): 1201–9. https://doi.org/10.3892/mmr.2016.5384.

Chen, Cho-Yi, Ryan W. Logan, Tianzhou Ma, David A. Lewis, George C. Tseng, Etienne Sibille, and Colleen A. McClung. 2016b. "Effects of Aging on Circadian Patterns of Gene Expression in the Human Prefrontal Cortex." *Proceedings of the National Academy of Sciences* 113 (1): 206–11. https://doi.org/10.1073/pnas.1508249112.

Chojnacki, Cezary, Ewa Walecka-Kapica, Aleksandra Błońska, Katarzyna Winczyk, Agnieszka Stępień, and Jan Chojnacki. 2016. "Serotonin and Melatonin Secretion in Postmenopausal Women with Eating Disorders." *Endokrynologia Polska* 67 (3): 299–304. https://doi.org/10.5603/EP.2016.0012.

Cipolla-Neto, J., F. G. Amaral, S. C. Afeche, D. X. Tan, and R. J. Reiter. 2014. "Melatonin, Energy Metabolism, and Obesity: A Review." *Journal of Pineal Research* 56 (4): 371–81. https://doi.org/10.1111/jpi.12137.

Colombo, Jucimara, João Marcos Wolf Maciel, Lívia Carvalho Ferreira, Renato Ferreira Da Silva, and Debora Aparecida Pires De Campos Zuccari. 2016. "Effects of Melatonin on HIF-1α and VEGF Expression and on the Invasive Properties of Hepatocarcinoma Cells." *Oncology Letters* 12 (1): 231–37. https://doi.org/10.3892/ol.2016.4605.

Coudert, Bruno, Christian Focan, Dominique Genet, Sylvie Giacchetti, Frédérique Cvickovic, Alberto Zambelli, Georges Fillet, et al. 2008. "A Randomized Multicenter Study of Optimal Circadian Time of Vinorelbine Combined with Chronomodulated 5-Fluorouracil in Pretreated Metastatic Breast Cancer Patients: EORTC Trial 05971." *Chronobiology International* 25 (5): 680–96. https://doi.org/10.1080/07420520802384036.

Crowley, Stephanie J., Christina Suh, Thomas A. Molina, Louis F. Fogg, Katherine M. Sharkey, and Mary A. Carskadon. 2016. "Estimating the Dim Light Melatonin Onset of Adolescents within a 6-h Sampling Window: The Impact of Sampling Rate and Threshold Method." *Sleep Medicine* 20 (April): 59–66. https://doi.org/10.1016/j.sleep.2015.11.019.

Culpepper, Larry, and Mark A. Wingertzahn. 2015. "Over-the-Counter Agents for the Treatment of Occasional Disturbed Sleep or Transient Insomnia: A Systematic Review of Efficacy and Safety." *The Primary Care Companion for CNS Disorders* 17 (6): 411–22. https://doi.org/10.4088/PCC.15r01798.

Dallmann, Robert, Alper Okyar, and Francis Lévi. 2016. "Dosing-Time Makes the Poison: Circadian Regulation and Pharmacotherapy." *Trends in Molecular Medicine* 22 (5): 430–45. https://doi.org/10.1016/j.molmed.2016.03.004.

Danilov, Andrei, and Julia Kurganova. 2016. "Melatonin in Chronic Pain Syndromes." *Pain and Therapy* 5 (1): 1–17. https://doi.org/10.1007/s40122-016-0049-y.

Davies, Sarah K., Joo Ern Ang, Victoria L. Revell, Ben Holmes, Anuska Mann, Francesca P. Robertson, Nanyi Cui, et al. 2014. "Effect of Sleep Deprivation on the Human Metabolome." *Proceedings of the National Academy of Sciences* 111 (29): 10761–66. https://doi.org/10.1073/pnas.1402663111.

Doddigarla, Zephy, Jamal Ahmad, and Iqbal Parwez. 2016. "Effect of Chromium Picolinate and Melatonin Either in Single or in a Combination in High Carbohydrate Diet-Fed Male Wistar Rats." *BioFactors (Oxford, England)* 42 (1): 106–14. https://doi.org/10.1002/biof.1253.

Dooley, James, Lei Tian, Susann Schonefeldt, Viviane Delghingaro-Augusto, Josselyn E. Garcia-Perez, Emanuela Pasciuto, Daniele Di Marino, et al. 2016. "Genetic Predisposition for Beta Cell Fragility Underlies Type 1 and Type 2 Diabetes." *Nature Genetics* 48 (5): 519–27. https://doi.org/10.1038/ng.3531.

Dowling, Glenna A., Robert L. Burr, Eus J. W. Van Someren, Erin M. Hubbard, Jay S. Luxenberg, Judy Mastick, and Bruce A. Cooper. 2008. "Melatonin and Bright-Light Treatment for Rest–Activity Disruption in Institutionalized Patients with Alzheimer's Disease." *Journal of the American Geriatrics Society* 56 (2): 239–46. https://doi.org/10.1111/j.1532-5415.2007.01543.x.

Dulong, Sandrine, Annabelle Ballesta, Alper Okyar, and Francis Lévi. 2015. "Identification of Circadian Determinants of Cancer Chronotherapy through In Vitro Chronopharmacology and Mathematical Modeling." *Molecular Cancer Therapeutics* 14 (9): 2154–64. https://doi.org/10.1158/1535-7163.MCT-15-0129.

Earnest, David J., Nichole Neuendorff, Jason Coffman, Amutha Selvamani, and Farida Sohrabji. 2016. "Sex Differences in the Impact of Shift Work Schedules on Pathological Outcomes in an Animal Model of Ischemic Stroke." *Endocrinology* 157 (7): 2836–43. https://doi.org/10.1210/en.2016-1130.

Emet, Mucaht, Halil Ozcan, Lutfu Ozel, Muhammed Yayla, Zekai Halici, and Ahmet Hacimuftuoglu. 2016. "A Review of Melatonin, Its Receptors and Drugs." *Eurasian Journal of Medicine* 48 (2): 135–41. https://doi.org/10.5152/eurasianjmed.2015.0267.

Enck, P., C. Kaiser, M. Felber, R. L. Riepl, A. Klauser, S. Klosterhalfen, and B. Otto. 2009. "Circadian Variation of Rectal Sensitivity and Gastrointestinal Peptides in Healthy Volunteers." *Neurogastroenterology & Motility* 21 (1): 52–58. https://doi.org/10.1111/j.1365-2982.2008.01182.x.

Erren, Thomas C., and Russel J. Reiter. 2015. "Melatonin: A Universal Time Messenger." *Neuro Endocrinology Letters* 36 (3): 187–92.

Esaki, Yuichi, Tsuyoshi Kitajima, Yasuhiro Ito, Shigefumi Koike, Yasumi Nakao, Akiko Tsuchiya, Marina Hirose, and Nakao Iwata. 2016. "Wearing Blue Light-Blocking Glasses in the Evening Advances Circadian Rhythms in the Patients with Delayed Sleep Phase Disorder: An Open-Label Trial." *Chronobiology International* 33 (8): 1037–44. https://doi.org/10.1080/07420 -528.2016.1194289.

Fanjul-Moles, María Luisa, and Germán Octavio López-Riquelme. 2016. "Relationship between Oxidative Stress, Circadian Rhythms, and AMD." *Oxidative Medicine and Cellular Longevity* (2016). https://doi .org/10.1155/2016/7420637.

Farriol, M., Y. Venereo, X. Orta, J. M. Castellanos, and T. Segovia-Silvestre. 2000. "In Vitro Effects of Melatonin on Cell Proliferation in a Colon Adenocarcinoma Line." *Journal of Applied Toxicology* 20 (1): 21–24. https://doi.org/10.1002 /(SICI)1099-1263(200001/02)20:1<21::AID-JAT623>3.0.CO;2-M.

Fauteck, J. D. 2001. "Melatonin: Is There a Rationale for the Clinical Use of This Hormone in Sleep Therapy?" *Zeitschrift Fur Arztliche Fortbildung Und Qualitatssicherung* 95 (1): 39–43.

Fauteck, J. D., J. Bockmann, T. M. Böckers, W. Wittkowski, R. Köhling, A. Lücke, H. Straub, et al. 1995. "Melatonin Reduces Low-Mg2+ Epileptiform Activity in Human Temporal Slices." *Experimental Brain Research* 107 (2): 321–25. https://doi.org/10.1007/BF00230052.

Fauteck, J. D., M. Dittgen, K. Farker, A. Hoffmann, H. Hoffmann, A. Lerchl, and W. Wittkowski. 1999. "Melatonin and Aging: Relevance for Clinical Approach?" *Journal of Endocrinological Investigation* 22 (10 Suppl): 90–91.

Fauteck, J. D., H. Schmidt, A. Lerchl, G. Kurlemann, and W. Wittkowski. 1999. "Melatonin in Epilepsy: First Results of Replacement Therapy and First Clinical Results." *Neurosignals* 8 (1–2): 105–10. https://doi .org/10.1159/000014577.

Fauteck, J. D., and I. Kusztrich. 2014. *Das Phytamin Prinzip. Besser länger leben mit Phytosto en und Hormonen.* Brandstätter: Verlag.

Fauteck, J. D., and T. M. Platzer. 2016. *Die Chrono Diät.* Brandstätter: Verlag.

Fauteck, Jan-Dirk, Alexander Lerchl, Markus Bergmann, Morten Møller, Franco Fraschini, Werner Wittkowski, and Bojidar Stankov. 1994. "The Adult Human Cerebellum Is a Target of the Neuroendocrine System

Involved in the Circadian Timing." *Neuroscience Letters* 179 (1): 60–64. https://doi.org/10.1016/0304-3940(94)90935-0.

Favero, Gaia, Luigi Fabrizio Rodella, Russel J. Reiter, and Rita Rezzani. 2014. "Melatonin and Its Atheroprotective Effects: A Review." *Molecular and Cellular Endocrinology* 382 (2): 926–37. https://doi.org/10.1016/j .mce.2013.11.016.

Fraschini, Franco, Russel J. Reiter, and Bojidar Stankov, eds. 1995. *The Pineal Gland and Its Hormones: Fundamentals and Clinical Perspectives.* Nato Science Series A: Springer US. https://www.springer.com/us /book/9781461357810.

Frye, Richard E., and Daniel A. Rossignol. 2016. "Identification and Treatment of Pathophysiological Comorbidities of Autism Spectrum Disorder to Achieve Optimal Outcomes." *Clinical Medicine Insights: Pediatrics* 10 (January): CMPed.S38337. https://doi.org/10.4137/CMPed .S38337.

Gao, Ling, Yi-Chao Zhao, Yan Liang, Xian-Hua Lin, Ya-Jing Tan, Dan-Dan Wu, Xin-Zhu Li, et al. 2016. "The Impaired Myocardial Ischemic Tolerance in Adult Offspring of Diabetic Pregnancy Is Restored by Maternal Melatonin Treatment." *Journal of Pineal Research* 61 (3): 340–52. https://doi.org/10.1111/jpi.12351.

Gapstur, Susan M., W. Ryan Diver, Victoria L. Stevens, Brian D. Carter, Lauren R. Teras, and Eric J. Jacobs. 2014. "Work Schedule, Sleep Duration, Insomnia, and Risk of Fatal Prostate Cancer." *American Journal of Preventive Medicine* 46 (3): S26–33. https://doi.org/10.1016/j .amepre.2013.10.033.

García-Mesa, Yoelvis, Lydia Giménez-Llort, Luis C. López, Carmen Venegas, Rosa Cristòfol, Germain Escames, Darío Acuña-Castroviejo, and Coral Sanfeliu. 2012. "Melatonin plus Physical Exercise Are Highly Neuroprotective in the 3xTg-AD Mouse." *Neurobiology of Aging* 33 (6): 1124.e13-1124.e29. https://doi.org/10.1016/j.neurobiolaging.2011.11.016.

Gelfand, Amy A., and Peter J. Goadsby. 2016. "The Role of Melatonin in the Treatment of Primary Headache Disorders." *Headache: The Journal of Head and Face Pain* 56 (8): 1257–66. https://doi.org/10.1111/head.12862.

Ghaeli, Padideh, Shaghayegh Vejdani, Atefeh Ariamanesh, and Azita Hajhossein Talasaz. 2015. "Effect of Melatonin on Cardiac Injury after Primary Percutaneous Coronary Intervention: A Randomized Controlled Trial." *Iranian Journal of Pharmaceutical Research: IJPR* 14 (3): 851–55.

Giskeødegård, Guro F., Sarah K. Davies, Victoria L. Revell, Hector Keun, and Debra J. Skene. 2015. "Diurnal Rhythms in the Human Urine Metabolome during Sleep and Total Sleep Deprivation." *Scientific Reports* 5 (October). https://doi.org/10.1038/srep14843.

Gonçalves, Andre Leite, Adriana Martini Ferreira, Reinaldo Teixeira Ribeiro, Eliova Zukerman, José Cipolla-Neto, and Mario Fernando Prieto Peres. 2016a. "Randomised Clinical Trial Comparing Melatonin 3 Mg, Amitriptyline 25 Mg and Placebo for Migraine Prevention." *Journal of Neurology, Neurosurgery, & Psychiatry* 87 (10): 1127–32. https://doi .org/10.1136/jnnp-2016-313458.

Gonçalves, Naiane do Nascimento, Jucimara Colombo, Juliana Ramos Lopes, Gabriela Bottaro Gelaleti, Marina Gobbe Moschetta, Nathália Martins Sonehara, Eva Hellmén, Caroline de Freitas Zanon, Sônia Maria Oliani, and Debora Aparecida Pires de Campos Zuccari. 2016b. "Effect of Melatonin in Epithelial Mesenchymal Transition Markers and Invasive Properties of Breast Cancer Stem Cells of Canine and Human Cell Lines." *PLOS ONE* 11 (3): e0150407. https://doi.org/10.1371/journal.pone.0150407.

Goswami, Soumik, and Chandana Haldar. 2015. "Melatonin as a Possible Antidote to UV Radiation Induced Cutaneous Damages and Immune-Suppression: An Overview." *Journal of Photochemistry and Photobiology B: Biology* 153 (December): 281–88. https://doi.org/10.1016/j .jphotobiol.2015.10.006.

Gramajo, A. L., G. E. Marquez, V. E. Torres, C. P. Juárez, R. E. Rosenstein, and J. D. Luna. 2015. "Therapeutic Benefit of Melatonin in Refractory Central Serous Chorioretinopathy." *Eye* 29 (8): 1036–45. https://doi.org/10.1038 /eye.2015.104.

Griebler, R., J. Anzenberger, and A. Eisenmann. 2014. *Herz-Kreislauf-Erkrankungen in Österreich: Angina Pectoris, Myokardinfarkt, ischämischer Schlaganfall, periphere arterielle Verschlusskrankheit. Epidemiologie und Prävention.* Wien: Bundesministerium für Gesundheit.

Gunn, Pippa J., Benita Middleton, Sarah K. Davies, Victoria L. Revell, and Debra J. Skene. 2016. "Sex Differences in the Circadian Profiles of Melatonin and Cortisol in Plasma and Urine Matrices under Constant Routine Conditions." *Chronobiology International* 33 (1): 39–50. https://doi .org/10.3109/07420528.2015.1112396.

Guo, Jing-Fang, and Bao-Zhen Yao. 2009. "Serum Melatonin Levels in Children with Epilepsy or Febrile Seizures." *Chinese Journal of Contemporary Pediatrics* 11 (4): 288–90.

Gutierrez, Daniel, and Joshua Arbesman. 2016. "Circadian Dysrhythmias, Physiological Aberrations, and the Link to Skin Cancer." *International Journal of Molecular Sciences* 17 (5): 621. https://doi.org/10.3390 /ijms17050621.

Gutierrez-Cuesta, J., M. Tajes, A. Jimenez, A. Camins, and M. Pallas. 2011. "Effects of Melatonin in the Brain of the Senescence-Accelerated Mice-Prone 8 (SAMP8) Model." *Revista De Neurologia* 52 (10): 618–22.

Gutierrez-Valdez, Ana Luisa, Verónica Anaya-Martínez, José Luis Ordoñez-Librado, Ricardo García-Ruiz, Carmen Torres-Esquivel, Montserrat Moreno-Rivera, Javier Sánchez-Betancourt, Enrique Montiel-Flores, and Maria Rosa Avila-Costa. 2012. "Effect of Chronic L-Dopa or Melatonin Treatments after Dopamine Deafferentation in Rats: Dyskinesia, Motor Performance, and Cytological Analysis." *International Scholarly Research Notices*. https://doi.org/10.5402/2012/360379.

Habtemariam, Solomon, Maria Daglia, Antoni Sureda, Zeliha Selamoglu, Mehmet Fuat Gulhan, and Seyed Mohammad Nabavi. 2017. "Melatonin and Respiratory Diseases: A Review." *Current Topics in Medicinal Chemistry* 17 (4): 467–88. http://www.eurekaselect.com/145042/article.

Hansen, M. V., A. K. Danielsen, I. Hageman, J. Rosenberg, and I. Gögenur. 2014. "The Therapeutic or Prophylactic Effect of Exogenous Melatonin against Depression and Depressive Symptoms: A Systematic Review and Meta-Analysis." *European Neuropsychopharmacology* 24 (11): 1719–28. https://doi.org/10.1016/j.euroneuro.2014.08.008.

Hardeland, Rüdiger. 2013. "Chronobiology of Melatonin beyond the Feedback to the Suprachiasmatic Nucleus—Consequences to Melatonin Dysfunction." *International Journal of Molecular Sciences* 14 (3): 5817–41. https://doi.org/10.3390/ijms14035817.

Harpsøe, Nathja Groth, Lars Peter Holst Andersen, Ismail Gögenur, and Jacob Rosenberg. 2015. "Clinical Pharmacokinetics of Melatonin: A Systematic Review." *European Journal of Clinical Pharmacology* 71 (8): 901–9. https://doi.org/10.1007/s00228-015-1873-4.

He, Changjiu, Jing Wang, Zhenzhen Zhang, Minghui Yang, Yu Li, Xiuzhi Tian, Teng Ma, et al. 2016. "Mitochondria Synthesize Melatonin to Ameliorate Its Function and Improve Mice Oocyte's Quality under in Vitro Conditions." *International Journal of Molecular Sciences* 17 (6): 939. https://doi.org/10.3390/ijms17060939.

Hermida, Ramón C., Diana E. Ayala, Artemio Mojón, and José R. Fernández. 2016. "Sleep-Time BP: Prognostic Marker of Type 2 Diabetes and Therapeutic Target for Prevention." *Diabetologia* 59 (2): 244–54. https://doi.org/10.1007/s00125-015-3748-8.

Hevia, David, Pedro González-Menéndez, Isabel Quiros-González, Ana Miar, Aida Rodríguez-García, Dun-Xian Tan, Russel J. Reiter, Juan C. Mayo, and Rosa M. Sainz. 2015. "Melatonin Uptake through Glucose Transporters: A New Target for Melatonin Inhibition of Cancer." *Journal of Pineal Research* 58 (2): 234–50. https://doi.org/10.1111/jpi.12210.

Hill, Steven M., Victoria P. Belancio, Robert T. Dauchy, Shulin Xiang, Samantha Brimer, Lulu Mao, Adam Hauch, et al. 2015. "Melatonin: An Inhibitor of Breast Cancer." *Endocrine-Related Cancer* 22 (3): R183–204. https://doi.org/10.1530/ERC-15-0030.

Hirsch-Rodriguez, Eric, Marta Imbesi, Radmila Manev, Tolga Uz, and Hari Manev. 2007. "The Pattern of Melatonin Receptor Expression in the Brain May Influence Antidepressant Treatment." *Medical Hypotheses* 69 (1): 120–24. https://doi.org/10.1016/j.mehy.2006.11.012.

Hoebert, Michel, Kristiaan B. Van Der Heijden, Ingeborg M. Van Geijlswijk, and Marcel G. Smits. 2009. "Long-Term Follow-up of Melatonin Treatment in Children with ADHD and Chronic Sleep Onset Insomnia." *Journal of Pineal Research* 47 (1): 1–7. https://doi.org/10.1111/j.1600-079X.2009.00681.x.

Hofstra-van Oostveen, Wytske A., and Al W. de Weerd. 2012. "Seizures, Epilepsy, and Circadian Rhythms." *Sleep Medicine Clinics* 7 (1): 99–104. https://doi.org/10.1016/j.jsmc.2011.12.005.

Hussain, Saad A., Haitham M. Khadim, Ban H. Khalaf, Sajida H. Ismail, Khalid I. Hussein, and Ahmed S. Sahib. 2006. "Effects of Melatonin and Zinc on Glycemic Control in Type 2 Diabetic Patients Poorly Controlled with Metformin." *Saudi Medical Journal* 27 (10): 1483–88.

Innominato, Pasquale F., Véronique P. Roche, Oxana G. Palesh, Ayhan Ulusakarya, David Spiegel, and Francis A. Lévi. 2014. "The Circadian Timing System in Clinical Oncology." *Annals of Medicine* 46 (4): 191–207. https://doi.org/10.3109/07853890.2014.916990.

Irwin, Michael R., Richard Olmstead, and Judith E. Carroll. 2016. "Sleep Disturbance, Sleep Duration, and Inflammation: A Systematic Review and Meta-Analysis of Cohort Studies and Experimental Sleep Deprivation." *Biological Psychiatry* 80 (1): 40–52. https://doi.org/10.1016/j.biopsych.2015.05.014.

Jain, Sejal V., Paul S. Horn, Narong Simakajornboon, Dean W. Beebe, Katherine Holland, Anna W. Byars, and Tracy A. Glauser. 2015. "Melatonin Improves Sleep in Children with Epilepsy: A Randomized, Double-Blind, Crossover Study." *Sleep Medicine* 16 (5): 637–44. https://doi.org/10.1016/j.sleep.2015.01.005.

Jehan, Shazia, Alina Masters-Isarilov, Idoko Salifu, Ferdinand Zizi, Jean-Louis Girardin, Seithikurippu R. Pandi-Perumal, Ravi Gupta, Amnon Brzezinski, and Samy I. McFarlane. 2015. "Sleep Disorders in Postmenopausal Women." *Journal of Sleep Disorders & Therapy* 4 (5). https://doi.org/10.4172/2167-0277.1000212.

Jockers, R., P. Maurice, J. A. Boutin, and P. Delagrange. 2008. "Melatonin Receptors, Heterodimerization, Signal Transduction and Binding Sites: What's New?" *British Journal of Pharmacology* 154 (6): 1182–95. https://doi.org/10.1038/bjp.2008.184.

Jockers, Ralf, Philippe Delagrange, Margarita L. Dubocovich, Regina P. Markus, Nicolas Renault, Gianluca Tosini, Erika Cecon, and Darius P. Zlotos. 2016. "Update on Melatonin Receptors: IUPHAR Review 20."

British Journal of Pharmacology 173 (18): 2702–25. https://doi.org/10.1111/bph.13536.

Johnston, Jonathan D., and Debra J. Skene. 2015. "Regulation of Mammalian Neuroendocrine Physiology and Rhythms by Melatonin." *Journal of Endocrinology* 226 (2): T187–98. https://doi.org/10.1530/JOE-15-0119.

Juszczak, Kajetan, and Tomasz Drewa. 2016. "The Multiple Biological Action Potential of Melatonin—Is Melatonin, Mitochondria and the Ischemic/Reperfusion Injury Relationship Essential in the Pathogenesis of Obstructive Nephropathy?" *Central European Journal of Urology* 69 (2): 231–32. https://doi.org/10.5173/ceju.2016.852.

Kalaria, R. N. 2012. "Risk Factors and Neurodegenerative Mechanisms in Stroke Related Dementia." *Panminerva Medica* 54 (3): 139–48.

Kallistratos, M. 2015. "Midday Naps Associated with Reduced Blood Pressure and Fewer Medications." https://www.escardio.org/The-ESC/Press-Office/Press-releases/Midday-naps-associated-with-reduced-blood-pressure-and-fewer-medications.

Kamal, Maud, Florence Gbahou, Jean-Luc Guillaume, Avais M. Daulat, Abla Benleulmi-Chaachoua, Marine Luka, Patty Chen, et al. 2015. "Convergence of Melatonin and Serotonin (5-HT) Signaling at MT2/5-HT2C Receptor Heteromers." *Journal of Biological Chemistry* 290 (18): 11537–46. https://doi.org/10.1074/jbc.M114.559542.

Karami, Zohre, Rostam Golmohammadi, Ahmad Heidaripahlavian, Jalal Poorolajal, and Rashid Heidarimoghadam. 2016. "Effect of Daylight on Melatonin and Subjective General Health Factors in Elderly People." *Iranian Journal of Public Health* 45 (5): 636–43.

Karatsoreos, Ilia N. 2014. "Links between Circadian Rhythms and Psychiatric Disease." *Frontiers in Behavioral Neuroscience* 8. https://doi.org/10.3389/fnbeh.2014.00162.

Keis, Oliver, Hannah Helbig, Judith Streb, and Katrin Hille. 2014. "Influence of Blue-Enriched Classroom Lighting on Students' Cognitive Performance." *Trends in Neuroscience and Education* 3 (3): 86–92. https://doi.org/10.1016/j.tine.2014.09.001.

Keshet-Sitton, Atalya, Keren Or-Chen, Sara Yitzhak, Ilana Tzabary, and Abraham Haim. 2016. "Can Avoiding Light at Night Reduce the Risk of Breast Cancer?" *Integrative Cancer Therapies* 15 (2): 145–52. https://doi.org/10.1177/1534735415618787.

Khorsand, Marjan, Masoumeh Akmali, Sahab Sharzad, and Mojtaba Beheshtitabar. 2016. "Melatonin Reduces Cataract Formation and Aldose Reductase Activity in Lenses of Streptozotocin-Induced Diabetic Rat." *Iranian Journal of Medical Sciences* 41 (4): 305–13.

Kiss, Zsofia, and Paramita M. Ghosh. 2016. "Circadian Rhythmicity and the Influence of 'Clock' Genes on Prostate Cancer." *Endocrine-Related Cancer* 23 (11): T123–34. https://doi.org/10.1530/ERC-16-0366.

Klaffke, S., and J. Staedt. 2006. "Sundowning and Circadian Rhythm Disorders in Dementia." *Acta Neurologica Belgica* 106 (4): 168–75.

Kloog, Itai, Abraham Haim, Richard G. Stevens, and Prof. Boris A. Portnov. 2009. "Global Co-Distribution of Light at Night (LAN) and Cancers of Prostate, Colon, and Lung in Men." *Chronobiology International* 26 (1): 108–25. https://doi.org/10.1080/07420520802694020.

Knight, Julia A., Suzanne Thompson, Janet M. Raboud, and Barry R. Hoffman. 2005. "Light and Exercise and Melatonin Production in Women." *American Journal of Epidemiology* 162 (11): 1114–22. https://doi.org/10.1093/aje/kwi327.

Kolev, P., P. Kumanov, A. Caronno, J. D. Fauteck, and B. M. Stankov. 2011. "Melatonina a rilascio controllato: Nuovi aspetti dell'utilizzo nell'uomo." *L'integratore nutrizionale* 14 (1).

Korkmaz, Ahmet, Shuran Ma, Turgut Topal, Sergio Rosales-Corral, Dun-Xian Tan, and Russel J. Reiter. 2012. "Glucose: A Vital Toxin and Potential Utility of Melatonin in Protecting against the Diabetic State." *Molecular and Cellular Endocrinology* 349 (2): 128–37. https://doi.org/10.1016/j.mce.2011.10.013.

Kumar, A. M., F. Tims, D. G. Cruess, M. J. Mintzer, G. Ironson, D. Loewenstein, R. Cattan, J. B. Fernandez, C. Eisdorfer, and M. Kumar. 1999. "Music Therapy Increases Serum Melatonin Levels in Patients with Alzheimer's Disease." *Alternative Therapies in Health and Medicine* 5 (6): 49–57.

Kunz, D. 2012. "Melatonin taktet die innere Uhr neu." *Neurologie and Psychiatrie* 14 (1).

Kunz, D. 2006. *Melatonin und Schlaf-Wach Regulation*. Berlin: Habilitationsschri.

Kurdi, Madhuri S., and Sindhu Priya Muthukalai. 2016. "The Efficacy of Oral Melatonin in Improving Sleep in Cancer Patients with Insomnia: A Randomized Double-Blind Placebo-Controlled Study." *Indian Journal of Palliative Care* 22 (3): 295. https://doi.org/10.4103/0973-1075.185039.

Lam, Raymond W., Anthony J. Levitt, Robert D. Levitan, Erin E. Michalak, Amy H. Cheung, Rachel Morehouse, Rajamannar Ramasubbu, Lakshmi N. Yatham, and Edwin M. Tam. 2016. "Efficacy of Bright Light Treatment, Fluoxetine, and the Combination in Patients with Nonseasonal Major Depressive Disorder: A Randomized Clinical Trial." *JAMA Psychiatry* 73 (1): 56–63. https://doi.org/10.1001/jamapsychiatry.2015.2235.

Lange, Tanja, Stoyan Dimitrov, and Jan Born. 2010. "Effects of Sleep and Circadian Rhythm on the Human Immune System." *Annals of the New*

York Academy of Sciences 1193 (1): 48–59. https://doi.org/10.1111 /j.1749-6632.2009.05300.x.

Lanoix, Dave, Pascale Guérin, and Cathy Vaillancourt. 2012. "Placental Melatonin Production and Melatonin Receptor Expression Are Altered in Preeclampsia: New Insights into the Role of This Hormone in Pregnancy." *Journal of Pineal Research* 53 (4): 417–25. https://doi .org/10.1111/j.1600-079X.2012.01012.x.

Lauretti, E., A. Di Meco, S. Merali, and D. Praticò. 2016. "Circadian Rhythm Dysfunction: A Novel Environmental Risk Factor for Parkinson's Disease." *Molecular Psychiatry* 22 (2): 280–86. https://doi.org/10.1038 /mp.2016.47.

Leclercq, Sophie, Paul Forsythe, and John Bienenstock. 2016. "Posttraumatic Stress Disorder: Does the Gut Microbiome Hold the Key?" *Canadian Journal of Psychiatry* 61 (4): 204–13. https://doi .org/10.1177/0706743716635535.

Leheste, Joerg R., and German Torres. 2015. "Resveratrol: Brain Effects on SIRT1, GPR50 and Photoperiodic Signaling." *Frontiers in Molecular Neuroscience* 8. https://doi.org/10.3389/fnmol.2015.00061.

Leonardi, Giulia Costanza, Venerando Rapisarda, Andrea Marconi, Aurora Scalisi, Francesca Catalano, Lidia Proietti, Salvo Travali, Massimo Libra, and Concettina Fenga. 2012. "Correlation of the Risk of Breast Cancer and Disruption of the Circadian Rhythm (Review)." *Oncology Reports* 28 (2): 418–28. https://doi.org/10.3892/or.2012.1839.

Letra-Vilela, Ricardo, Ana María Sánchez-Sánchez, Ana Maia Rocha, Vanesa Martin, Joana Branco-Santos, Noelia Puente-Moncada, Mariana Santa-Marta, et al. 2016. "Distinct Roles of N-Acetyl and 5-Methoxy Groups in the Antiproliferative and Neuroprotective Effects of Melatonin." *Molecular and Cellular Endocrinology* 434 (October): 238–49. https://doi .org/10.1016/j.mce.2016.07.012.

Lewy, Alfred J., and Robert L. Sack. 1989. "The Dim Light Melatonin Onset as a Marker for Orcadian Phase Position." *Chronobiology International* 6 (1): 93–102. https://doi.org/10.3109/07420528909059144.

Li, Jun Z., Blynn G. Bunney, Fan Meng, Megan H. Hagenauer, David M. Walsh, Marquis P. Vawter, Simon J. Evans, et al. 2013. "Circadian Patterns of Gene Expression in the Human Brain and Disruption in Major Depressive Disorder." *Proceedings of the National Academy of Sciences* 110 (24): 9950–55. https://doi.org/10.1073/pnas.1305814110.

Li, Weimin, Mengdi Fan, Yina Chen, Qian Zhao, Caiyun Song, Ye Yan, Yin Jin, Zhiming Huang, Chunjing Lin, and Jiansheng Wu. 2015. "Melatonin Induces Cell Apoptosis in AGS Cells Through the Activation of JNK and P38 MAPK and the Suppression of Nuclear Factor-Kappa B: A Novel

Therapeutic Implication for Gastric Cancer." *Cellular Physiology and Biochemistry* 37 (6): 2323–38. https://doi.org/10.1159/000438587.

Lima, Eliângela, Francisco R. Cabral, Esper A. Cavalheiro, Maria da Graça Naffah-Mazzacoratti, and Débora Amado. 2011. "Melatonin Administration after Pilocarpine-Induced Status Epilepticus: A New Way to Prevent or Attenuate Postlesion Epilepsy?" *Epilepsy & Behavior* 20 (4): 607–12. https://doi.org/10.1016/j.yebeh.2011.01.018.

Lin, Yu-Kai, Guan-Yu Lin, Jiunn-Tay Lee, Meei-Shyuan Lee, Chia-Kuang Tsai, Yu-Wei Hsu, Yu-Zhen Lin, Yi-Chien Tsai, and Fu-Chi Yang. 2016. "Associations Between Sleep Quality and Migraine Frequency: A Cross -Sectional Case-Control Study." *Medicine* 95 (17). https://doi.org/10.1097 /MD.0000000000003554.

Lissoni, P. 2002. "Is There a Role for Melatonin in Supportive Care?" *Supportive Care in Cancer* 10 (2): 110–16. https://doi.org/10.1007 /s005200100281.

Lissoni, P. 2007. "Biochemotherapy with Standard Chemotherapies plus the Pineal Hormone Melatonin in the Treatment of Advanced Solid Neoplasms." *Pathologie Biologie* 55 (3): 201–4. https://doi.org/10.1016/j .patbio.2006.12.025.

Lissoni, P., S. Barni, M. Mandalà, A. Ardizzoia, F. Paolorossi, M. Vaghi, R. Longarini, F. Malugani, and G. Tancini. 1999. "Decreased Toxicity and Increased Efficacy of Cancer Chemotherapy Using the Pineal Hormone Melatonin in Metastatic Solid Tumour Patients with Poor Clinical Status." *European Journal of Cancer* 35 (12): 1688–92. https://doi.org/10.1016 /S0959-8049(99)00159-8.

Loy, F., M. Isola, R. Isola, P. Solinas, M. A. Lilliu, R. Puxeddu, and J. Ekstrom. 2015. "Ultrastructural Evidence of a Secretory Role for Melatonin in the Human Parotid Gland." *Journal of Physiology and Pharmacology* 66 (6): 847–53.

Ma, C., L. X. Li, Y. Zhang, C. Xiang, T. Ma, Z. Q. Ma, and Z. P. Zhang. 2015. "Protective and Sensitive Effects of Melatonin Combined with Adriamycin on ER+ (Estrogen Receptor) Breast Cancer." *European Journal of Gynaecological Oncology* 36 (2): 197–202.

Mack, Josiel Mileno, Marissa Giovanna Schamne, Tuane Bazanella Sampaio, Renata Aparecida Nedel Pértile, Pedro Augusto Carlos Magno Fernandes, Regina P. Markus, and Rui Daniel Prediger. 2016. "Melatoninergic System in Parkinson's Disease: From Neuroprotection to the Management of Motor and Nonmotor Symptoms." *Oxidative Medicine and Cellular Longevity*. https://doi.org/10.1155/2016/3472032.

Madsen, Helle Østergaard, Henrik Dam, and Ida Hageman. 2016a. "High Prevalence of Seasonal Affective Disorder among Persons with Severe

Visual Impairment." *British Journal of Psychiatry* 208 (1): 56–61. https://doi.org/10.1192/bjp.bp.114.162354.

Madsen, Michael Tvilling, Melissa Voigt Hansen, Lærke Toftegård Andersen, Ida Hageman, Lars Simon Rasmussen, Susanne Bokmand, Jacob Rosenberg, and Ismail Gögenur. 2016b. "Effect of Melatonin on Sleep in the Perioperative Period after Breast Cancer Surgery: A Randomized, Double-Blind, Placebo-Controlled Trial." *Journal of Clinical Sleep Medicine* 12 (02): 225–33. https://doi.org/10.5664/jcsm.5490.

Mahdi, Abbas Ali, Ghizal Fatima, Siddhartha Kumar Das, and Nar Singh Verma. 2011. "Abnormality of Circadian Rhythm of Serum Melatonin and Other Biochemical Parameters in Fibromyalgia Syndrome." *Indian Journal of Biochemistry & Biophysics* 48 (2): 82–87.

Mahmood, Danish, Bala Yauri Muhammad, Mahfoudh Alghani, Jamir Anwar, Nasra el-Lebban, and Mohammad Haider. 2016. "Advancing Role of Melatonin in the Treatment of Neuropsychiatric Disorders." *Egyptian Journal of Basic and Applied Sciences* 3 (3): 203–18. https://doi.org/10.1016/j.ejbas.2016.07.001.

Manni, Raffaele, Roberto De Icco, Riccardo Cremascoli, Giulia Ferrera, Francesca Furia, Elena Zambrelli, Maria Paola Canevini, and Michele Terzaghi. 2016. "Circadian Phase Typing in Idiopathic Generalized Epilepsy: Dim Light Melatonin Onset and Patterns of Melatonin Secretion—Semicurve Findings in Adult Patients." *Epilepsy & Behavior* 61 (August): 132–37. https://doi.org/10.1016/j.yebeh.2016.05.019.

Mao, Lulu, Robert T. Dauchy, David E. Blask, Erin M. Dauchy, Lauren M. Slakey, Samantha Brimer, Lin Yuan, et al. 2016. "Melatonin Suppression of Aerobic Glycolysis (Warburg Effect), Survival Signalling and Metastasis in Human Leiomyosarcoma." *Journal of Pineal Research* 60 (2): 167–77. https://doi.org/10.1111/jpi.12298.

Martínez-Águila, Alejandro, Begoña Fonseca, María J. Pérez de Lara, and Jesús Pintor. 2016. "Effect of Melatonin and 5-Methoxycarbonylamino-N-Acetyltryptamine on the Intraocular Pressure of Normal and Glaucomatous Mice." *Journal of Pharmacology and Experimental Therapeutics* 357 (2): 293–99. https://doi.org/10.1124/jpet.115.231456.

Matsumura, Ritsuko, Koichi Node, and Makoto Akashi. 2016. "Estimation Methods for Human Circadian Phase by Use of Peripheral Tissues." *Hypertension Research* 39 (9): 623–27. https://doi.org/10.1038/hr.2016.68.

Mayo, Juan C., David Hevia, Isabel Quiros-Gonzalez, Aida Rodriguez-Garcia, Pedro Gonzalez-Menendez, Vanesa Cepas, Iván Gonzalez-Pola, and Rosa M. Sainz. 2017. "IGFBP3 and MAPK/ERK Signaling Mediates Melatonin-Induced Antitumor Activity in Prostate Cancer." *Journal of Pineal Research* 62 (1): e12373. https://doi.org/10.1111/jpi.12373.

McMahon, Brenda, Sofie B. Andersen, Martin K. Madsen, Liv V. Hjordt, Ida Hageman, Henrik Dam, Claus Svarer, et al. 2016. "Seasonal Difference in Brain Serotonin Transporter Binding Predicts Symptom Severity in Patients with Seasonal Affective Disorder." *Brain* 139 (5): 1605–14. https://doi.org/10.1093/brain/aww043.

McMullan, Ciaran J., Gary C. Curhan, Eva S. Schernhammer, and John P. Forman. 2013. "Association of Nocturnal Melatonin Secretion with Insulin Resistance in Nondiabetic Young Women." *American Journal of Epidemiology* 178 (2): 231–38. https://doi.org/10.1093/aje/kws470.

Meliska, Charles J., Luis F. Martínez, Ana M. López, Diane L. Sorenson, Sara Nowakowski, Daniel F. Kripke, Jeffrey Elliott, and Barbara L. Parry. 2013. "Antepartum Depression Severity Is Increased During Seasonally Longer Nights: Relationship to Melatonin and Cortisol Timing and Quantity." *Chronobiology International* 30 (9): 1160–73. https://doi.org/10.3109/07420 -528.2013.808652.

Mendoza-Mendieta, María Elena, and Ana Aurora Lorenzo-Mejía. 2016. "Associated Depression in Pseudophakic Patients with Intraocular Lens with and without Chromophore." *Clinical Ophthalmology*. https://doi .org/10.2147/OPTH.S95212.

Michael, Alicia K., Stacy L. Harvey, Patrick J. Sammons, Amanda P. Anderson, Hema M. Kopalle, Alison H. Banham, and Carrie L. Partch. 2015. "Cancer/Testis Antigen PASD1 Silences the Circadian Clock." *Molecular Cell* 58 (5): 743–54. https://doi.org/10.1016/j.molcel.2015.03.031.

Morris, Christopher J., Jessica N. Yang, Joanna I. Garcia, Samantha Myers, Isadora Bozzi, Wei Wang, Orfeu M. Buxton, Steven A. Shea, and Frank A. J. L. Scheer. 2015. "Endogenous Circadian System and Circadian Misalignment Impact Glucose Tolerance via Separate Mechanisms in Humans." *Proceedings of the National Academy of Sciences* 112 (17): E2225–34. https://doi.org/10.1073/pnas.1418955112.

Mundey, Kavita, Susan Benloucif, Krisztina Harsanyi, Margarita L. Dubocovich, and Phyllis C. Zee. 2005. "Phase-Dependent Treatment of Delayed Sleep Phase Syndrome with Melatonin." *Sleep* 28 (10): 1271–78. https://doi.org/10.1093/sleep/28.10.1271.

Nagtegaal, J. E., G. A. Kerkhof, M. G. Smits, A. C. Swart, and Y. G. Van Der Meer. 1998. "Delayed Sleep Phase Syndrome: A Placebo-Controlled Cross-over Study on the Effects of Melatonin Administered Five Hours before the Individual Dim Light Melatonin Onset." *Journal of Sleep Research* 7 (2): 135–43. https://doi.org/10.1046/j.1365-2869.1998.00102.x.

Najjar, Raymond P., and Jamie M. Zeitzer. 2016. "Temporal Integration of Light Flashes by the Human Circadian System." *Journal of Clinical Investigation* 126 (3): 938–47. https://doi.org/10.1172/JCI82306.

Nakamura, Yasuhiko, Hiroshi Tamura, Shiro Kashida, Hisako Takayama, Yoshiaki Yamagata, Ayako Karube, Norihiro Sugino, and Hiroshi Kato. 2001. "Changes of Serum Melatonin Level and Its Relationship to Feto-Placental Unit during Pregnancy." *Journal of Pineal Research* 30 (1): 29–33. https://doi.org/10.1034/j.1600-079X.2001.300104.x.

Nooshinfar, Elaheh, Ava Safaroghli-Azar, Davood Bashash, and Mohammad Esmaeil Akbari. 2017. "Melatonin, an Inhibitory Agent in Breast Cancer." *Breast Cancer* 24 (1): 42–51. https://doi.org/10.1007/s12282-016-0690-7.

Ocmen, Elvan, Hale Aksu Erdost, Leyla S. Duru, Pinar Akan, Dilek Cimrin, and Ali N. Gokmen. 2016. "Effect of Day/Night Administration of Three Different Inhalational Anesthetics on Melatonin Levels in Rats." *Kaohsiung Journal of Medical Sciences* 32 (6): 302–5. https://doi.org/10.1016/j.kjms.2016.04.016.

Ortiz-Tudela, E., A. Mteyrek, A. Ballesta, P. F. Innominato, and F. Lévi. 2013. "Cancer Chronotherapeutics: Experimental, Theoretical, and Clinical Aspects." In *Circadian Clocks*, edited by Achim Kramer and Martha Merrow, 261–88. Handbook of Experimental Pharmacology. Berlin, Heidelberg: Springer Berlin Heidelberg. https://doi.org/10.1007/978-3-642-25950-0_11.

Owino, Sharon, Susana Contreras-Alcantara, Kenkichi Baba, and Gianluca Tosini. 2016. "Melatonin Signaling Controls the Daily Rhythm in Blood Glucose Levels Independent of Peripheral Clocks." *PLOS ONE* 11 (1): e0148214. https://doi.org/10.1371/journal.pone.0148214.

Ozsoy, Mustafa, Yucel Gonul, Ziya Taner Ozkececi, Ahmet Bali, Ruchan Bahadir Celep, Ahmet Koçak, Fahri Adali, Murat Tosun, and Sefa Celik. 2016. "The Protective Effect of Melatonin on Remote Organ Liver Ischemia and Reperfusion Injury Following Aortic Clamping." *Annali Italiani Di Chirurgia* 87: 271–79.

Ozturk, Hulya, Hayrettin Öztürk, Yusuf Yagmur, and Ali Kemal Uzunlar. 2006. "Effects of Melatonin Administration on Intestinal Adaptive Response After Massive Bowel Resection in Rats." *Digestive Diseases and Sciences* 51 (2): 333–37. https://doi.org/10.1007/s10620-006-3134-y.

Paine, Sarah-Jane, and Philippa H. Gander. 2016. "Differences in Circadian Phase and Weekday/Weekend Sleep Patterns in a Sample of Middle-Aged Morning Types and Evening Types." *Chronobiology International* 33 (8): 1009–17. https://doi.org/10.1080/07420528.2016.1192187.

Pandi-Perumal, Seithikurippu R., Ahmed S. BaHammam, Gregory M. Brown, D. Warren Spence, Vijay K. Bharti, Charanjit Kaur, Rüdiger Hardeland, and Daniel P. Cardinali. 2013. "Melatonin Antioxidative Defense: Therapeutic Implications for Aging and Neurodegenerative Processes." *Neurotoxicity Research* 23 (3): 267–300. https://doi.org/10.1007/s12640-012-9337-4.

Papagiannakopoulos, Thales, Matthew R. Bauer, Shawn M. Davidson, Megan Heimann, Lakshmipriya Subbaraj, Arjun Bhutkar, Jordan Bartlebaugh, Matthew G. Vander Heiden, and Tyler Jacks. 2016. "Circadian Rhythm Disruption Promotes Lung Tumorigenesis." *Cell Metabolism* 24 (2): 324–31. https://doi.org/10.1016/j.cmet.2016.07.001.

Parandavar, Nehleh, Khadijeh Abdali, Sara Keshtgar, Maasoumeh Emamghoreishi, and Seddegheh Amooee. 2014. "The Effect of Melatonin on Climacteric Symptoms in Menopausal Women; A Double-Blind, Randomized Controlled, Clinical Trial." *Iranian Journal of Public Health* 43 (10): 1405–16.

Paulose, Jiffin K., John M. Wright, Akruti G. Patel, and Vincent M. Cassone. 2016. "Human Gut Bacteria Are Sensitive to Melatonin and Express Endogenous Circadian Rhythmicity." *PLOS ONE* 11 (1): e0146643. https://doi.org/10.1371/journal.pone.0146643.

Pechanova, Olga, Ludovit Paulis, and Fedor Simko. 2014. "Peripheral and Central Effects of Melatonin on Blood Pressure Regulation." *International Journal of Molecular Sciences* 15 (10): 17920–37. https://doi.org/10.3390/ijms151017920.

Pei, Haifeng, Jin Du, Xiaofeng Song, Lei He, Yufei Zhang, Xiuchuan Li, Chenming Qiu, et al. 2016. "Melatonin Prevents Adverse Myocardial Infarction Remodeling via Notch1/Mfn2 Pathway." *Free Radical Biology and Medicine* 97 (August): 408–17. https://doi.org/10.1016/j.freeradbiomed.2016.06.015.

Pei, Zhong, S. F. Pang, and R. T. F. Cheung. 2002. "Pretreatment with Melatonin Reduces Volume of Cerebral Infarction in a Rat Middle Cerebral Artery Occlusion Stroke Model." *Journal of Pineal Research* 32 (3): 168–72. https://doi.org/10.1034/j.1600-079x.2002.10847.x.

Peschke, Elmar, Ina Bähr, and Eckhard Mühlbauer. 2015. "Experimental and Clinical Aspects of Melatonin and Clock Genes in Diabetes." *Journal of Pineal Research* 59 (1): 1–23. https://doi.org/10.1111/jpi.12240.

Pierpaoli, W., and W. Regelson. 1995. *The Melatonin Miracle.* New York: Simon and Schuster.

Pillittere, Donna, and Mike Miller. 2000. "Researchers Search for Link Between Circadian Rhythms, Breast Cancer." *Journal of the National Cancer Institute* 92 (9): 686–89. https://doi.org/10.1093/jnci/92.9.686.

Prather, Aric A., Denise Janicki-Deverts, Martica H. Hall, and Sheldon Cohen. 2015. "Behaviorally Assessed Sleep and Susceptibility to the Common Cold." *Sleep* 38 (9): 1353–59. https://doi.org/10.5665/sleep.4968.

Prosser, Rebecca A., and J. David Glass. 2015. "Assessing Ethanol's Actions in the Suprachiasmatic Circadian Clock Using in Vivo and in Vitro Approaches." *Alcohol,* Special Issue: Sleep, Circadian Rhythms and Alcohol, 49 (4): 321–39. https://doi.org/10.1016/j.alcohol.2014.07.016.

Qian, Jingyi, and Frank A. J. L. Scheer. 2016. "Circadian System and Glucose Metabolism: Implications for Physiology and Disease." *Trends in Endocrinology & Metabolism* 27 (5): 282–93. https://doi.org/10.1016/j.tem.2016.03.005.

Quigg, Mark. 2000. "Circadian Rhythms: Interactions with Seizures and Epilepsy." *Epilepsy Research* 42 (1): 43–55. https://doi.org/10.1016/S0920-1211(00)00157-1.

Radwan, P., B. Skrzydlo-Radomanska, K. Radwan-Kwiatek, B. Burak-Czapiuk, and J. Strzemecka. 2009. "Is Melatonin Involved in the Irritable Bowel Syndrome?" *Journal of Physiology and Pharmacology: An Official Journal of the Polish Physiological Society* 60, Suppl. 3 (October): 67–70.

Rasch, Björn, and Jan Born. 2013. "About Sleep's Role in Memory." *Physiological Reviews* 93 (2): 681–766. https://doi.org/10.1152/physrev.00032.2012.

Reiter, R. J., and J. Robinson. 1995. *Melatonin: Breakthrough Discoveries That Can Help You Combat Aging, Boost Your Immune System, Reduce Your Risk of Cancer and Heart Disease, Get a Better Night's Sleep.* New York: Bantam.

Reiter, Russel J., Hiroshi Tamura, Dun Xian Tan, and Xiao-Ying Xu. 2014b. "Melatonin and the Circadian System: Contributions to Successful Female Reproduction." *Fertility and Sterility* 102 (2): 321–28. https://doi.org/10.1016/j.fertnstert.2014.06.014.

Reiter, Russel J., Juan C. Mayo, Dun-Xian Tan, Rosa M. Sainz, Moises Alatorre-Jimenez, and Lilan Qin. 2016. "Melatonin as an Antioxidant: Under Promises but over Delivers." *Journal of Pineal Research* 61 (3): 253–78. https://doi.org/10.1111/jpi.12360.

Reiter, Russel J., Dun Xian Tan, Ahmet Korkmaz, and Sergio A. Rosales-Corral. 2014c. "Melatonin and Stable Circadian Rhythms Optimize Maternal, Placental and Fetal Physiology." *Human Reproduction Update* 20 (2): 293–307. https://doi.org/10.1093/humupd/dmt054.

Reiter, Russel J., Dun-Xian Tan, and Annia Galano. 2014a. "Melatonin: Exceeding Expectations." *Physiology* 29 (5): 325–33. https://doi.org/10.1152/physiol.00011.2014.

Reiter, Russel J., Dun-Xian Tan, and Annia Galano. 2014e. "Melatonin Reduces Lipid Peroxidation and Membrane Viscosity." *Frontiers in Physiology* 5. https://doi.org/10.3389/fphys.2014.00377.

Reiter, Russel J., Dun-Xian Tan, and Lorena Fuentes-Broto. 2010b. "Melatonin: A Multitasking Molecule." In *Progress in Brain Research*, edited by Luciano Martini, 181:127–51. Neuroendocrinology: The Normal Neuroendocrine System. Elsevier. https://doi.org/10.1016/S0079-6123(08)81008-4.

Reiter, Russel J., Dun-Xian Tan, Hiroshi Tamura, Maria Helena C. Cruz, and Lorena Fuentes-Broto. 2014d. "Clinical Relevance of Melatonin in Ovarian and Placental Physiology: A Review." *Gynecological Endocrinology* 30 (2): 83–89. https://doi.org/10.3109/09513590.2013.849238.

Reiter, Russel J., Dun-Xian Tan, Sergio D. Paredes, and Lorena Fuentes-Broto. 2010a. "Beneficial Effects of Melatonin in Cardiovascular Disease." *Annals of Medicine* 42 (4): 276–85. https://doi.org/10.3109/07853890903485748.

Reiter, Russel J., Dun-Xian Tan, Zhou Zhou, Maria Helena Coelho Cruz, Lorena Fuentes-Broto, and Annia Galano. 2015. "Phytomelatonin: Assisting Plants to Survive and Thrive." *Molecules* 20 (4): 7396–7437. https://doi.org/10.3390/molecules20047396.

Rivara, Silvia, Daniele Pala, Annalida Bedini, and Gilberto Spadoni. 2015. "Therapeutic Uses of Melatonin and Melatonin Derivatives: A Patent Review (2012 – 2014)." *Expert Opinion on Therapeutic Patents* 25 (4): 425–41. https://doi.org/10.1517/13543776.2014.1001739.

Rondanelli, Mariangela, Milena Anna Faliva, Simone Perna, and Neldo Antoniello. 2013. "Update on the Role of Melatonin in the Prevention of Cancer Tumorigenesis and in the Management of Cancer Correlates, Such as Sleep-Wake and Mood Disturbances: Review and Remarks." *Aging Clinical and Experimental Research* 25 (5): 499–510. https://doi.org/10.1007/s40520-013-0118-6.

Rosales-Corral, Sergio A., Dario Acuña-Castroviejo, Ana Coto-Montes, Jose A. Boga, Lucien C. Manchester, Lorena Fuentes-Broto, Ahmet Korkmaz, Shuran Ma, Dun-Xian Tan, and Russel J. Reiter. 2012. "Alzheimer's Disease: Pathological Mechanisms and the Beneficial Role of Melatonin." *Journal of Pineal Research* 52 (2): 167–202. https://doi.org/10.1111/j.1600-079X.2011.00937.x.

Rosen, Richard B., Dan-Ning Hu, Min Chen, Steven A. McCormick, Joseph Walsh, and Joan E. Roberts. 2012. "Effects of Melatonin and Its Receptor Antagonist on Retinal Pigment Epithelial Cells against Hydrogen Peroxide Damage." *Molecular Vision* 18: 1640–48.

Ruan, Guo-Xiang, Dao-Qi Zhang, Tongrong Zhou, Shin Yamazaki, and Douglas G. McMahon. 2006. "Circadian Organization of the Mammalian Retina." *Proceedings of the National Academy of Sciences* 103 (25): 9703–8. https://doi.org/10.1073/pnas.0601940103.

Rudic, R. Daniel. 2009. "Time Is of the Essence." *Circulation* 120 (17): 1714–21. https://doi.org/10.1161/CIRCULATIONAHA.109.853002.

Rutters, Femke, Sofie G. Lemmens, Tanja C. Adam, Marijke A. Bremmer, Petra J. Elders, Giel Nijpels, and Jacqueline M. Dekker. 2014. "Is Social Jetlag Associated with an Adverse Endocrine, Behavioral, and Cardiovascular Risk Profile?" *Journal of Biological Rhythms* 29 (5): 377–83. https://doi.org/10.1177/0748730414550199.

Sahar, Saurabh, and Paolo Sassone-Corsi. 2009. "Metabolism and Cancer: The Circadian Clock Connection." *Nature Reviews Cancer* 9 (12): 886–96. https://doi.org/10.1038/nrc2747.

Sánchez-Barceló, E. J., M. D. Mediavilla, D. X. Tan, and R. J. Reiter. 2010. "Clinical Uses of Melatonin: Evaluation of Human Trials." *Current Medicinal Chemistry* 17 (19): 2070–95. http://www.eurekaselect.com /71686/article.

Sánchez-Barceló, Emilio J., Maria D. Mediavilla, Carolina Alonso-Gonzalez, and Russel J. Reiter. 2012. "Melatonin Uses in Oncology: Breast Cancer Prevention and Reduction of the Side Effects of Chemotherapy and Radiation." *Expert Opinion on Investigational Drugs* 21 (6): 819–31. https: //doi.org/10.1517/13543784.2012.681045.

Santhi, Nayantara, Alpar S. Lazar, Patrick J. McCabe, June C. Lo, John A. Groeger, and Derk-Jan Dijk. 2016. "Sex Differences in the Circadian Regulation of Sleep and Waking Cognition in Humans." *Proceedings of the National Academy of Sciences* 113 (19): E2730–39. https://doi.org/10.1073 /pnas.1521637113.

Savaskan, Egemen, Mohammed A. Ayoub, Rivka Ravid, Debora Angeloni, Franco Fraschini, Fides Meier, Anne Eckert, Franz Müller-Spahn, and Ralf Jockers. 2005. "Reduced Hippocampal MT2 Melatonin Receptor Expression in Alzheimer's Disease." *Journal of Pineal Research* 38 (1): 10–16. https://doi.org/10.1111/j.1600-079X.2004.00169.x.

Scheer, Frank A. J. L., Christopher J. Morris, Joanna I. Garcia, Carolina Smales, Erin E. Kelly, Jenny Marks, Atul Malhotra, and Steven A. Shea. 2012. "Repeated Melatonin Supplementation Improves Sleep in Hypertensive Patients Treated with Beta-Blockers: A Randomized Controlled Trial." *Sleep* 35 (10): 1395–1402. https://doi.org/10.5665 /sleep.2122.

Scheer Frank A.J.L., Van Montfrans Gert A., van Someren Eus J.W., Mairuhu Gideon, and Buijs Ruud M. 2004. "Daily Nighttime Melatonin Reduces Blood Pressure in Male Patients With Essential Hypertension." *Hypertension* 43 (2): 192–97. https://doi.org/10.1161/01 .HYP.0000113293.15186.3b.

Scheuer, Cecilie, Hans-Christian Pommergaard, Jacob Rosenberg, and Ismail Gögenur. 2014. "Melatonin's Protective Effect against UV Radiation: A Systematic Review of Clinical and Experimental Studies." *Photodermatology, Photoimmunology & Photomedicine* 30 (4): 180–88. https://doi.org/10.1111/phpp.12080.

Scholtens, Rikie M., Barbara C. van Munster, Marijn F. van Kempen, and Sophia E. J. A. de Rooij. 2016. "Physiological Melatonin Levels in Healthy Older People: A Systematic Review." *Journal of Psychosomatic Research* 86 (July): 20–27. https://doi.org/10.1016/j.jpsychores.2016.05.005.

Schwichtenberg, A. J., and Beth A. Malow. 2015. "Melatonin Treatment in Children with Developmental Disabilities." *Sleep Medicine Clinics* 10 (2): 181–87. https://doi.org/10.1016/j.jsmc.2015.02.008.

Seabra, Maria de Lourdes V., Magda Bignotto, Luciano R. Pinto Jr., and Sergio Tufik. 2000. "Randomized, Double-Blind Clinical Trial, Controlled with Placebo, of the Toxicology of Chronic Melatonin Treatment." *Journal of Pineal Research* 29 (4): 193–200. https://doi.org/10.1034/j.1600-0633.2002.290401.x.

Seely, Dugald, Ping Wu, Heidi Fritz, Deborah A. Kennedy, Teresa Tsui, Andrew J. E. Seely, and Edward Mills. 2012. "Melatonin as Adjuvant Cancer Care with and Without Chemotherapy: A Systematic Review and Meta-Analysis of Randomized Trials." *Integrative Cancer Therapies* 11 (4): 293–303. https://doi.org/10.1177/1534735411425484.

Seifpanahi-Shabani, H., M. Abbasi, I. Salehi, Z. Yousefpour, and A. Zamani. 2016. "Long-Term Exposure to Extremely Low Frequency Electromagnetic Field and Melatonin Production by Blood Cells." *International Journal of Occupational and Environmental Medicine* 7 (3): 193–94. https://doi.org/10.15171/ijoem.2016.807.

Sharma, Shweta, Hemant Singh, Nabeel Ahmad, Priyanka Mishra, Archana Tiwari, Shweta Sharma, Hemant Singh, Nabeel Ahmad, Priyanka Mishra, and Archana Tiwari. 2015. "The Role of Melatonin in Diabetes: Therapeutic Implications." *Archives of Endocrinology and Metabolism* 59 (5): 391–99. https://doi.org/10.1590/2359-3997000000098.

Shechter, Ari, and Diane B. Boivin. 2010. "Sleep, Hormones, and Circadian Rhythms throughout the Menstrual Cycle in Healthy Women and Women with Premenstrual Dysphoric Disorder." *International Journal of Endocrinology.* https://doi.org/10.1155/2010/259345.

Shenshen, Yan, Wang Minshu, Yuan Qing, Liu Yang, Zhai Suodi, and Wang Wei. 2016. "The Effect of Cataract Surgery on Salivary Melatonin and Sleep Quality in Aging People." *Chronobiology International* 33 (8): 1064–72. https://doi.org/10.1080/07420528.2016.1197234.

Sipilä, Jussi O., Jori Ruuskanen, Päivi Rautava, and Ville Kytö. 2016. "Daylight Saving Time Transitions, Incidence and In-Hospital Mortality of Ischemic Stroke (S32.008)." *Neurology* 86 (16 Supplement): S32.008.

Skene, Debra J., and Josephine Arendt. 2007. "Circadian Rhythm Sleep Disorders in the Blind and Their Treatment with Melatonin." *Sleep Medicine*, Circadian Rhythms in Sleep Medicine, 8 (6): 651–55. https://doi.org/10.1016/j.sleep.2006.11.013.

Slominski, Andrzej T., Konrad Kleszczyński, Igor Semak, Zorica Janjetovic, Michał A. Żmijewski, Tae-Kang Kim, Radomir M. Slominski, Russel J. Reiter, and Tobias W. Fischer. 2014. "Local Melatoninergic System as the

Protector of Skin Integrity." *International Journal of Molecular Sciences* 15 (10): 17705–32. https://doi.org/10.3390/ijms151017705.

Slominski, Radomir M., Russel J. Reiter, Natalia Schlabritz-Loutsevitch, Rennolds S. Ostrom, and Andrzej T. Slominski. 2012. "Melatonin Membrane Receptors in Peripheral Tissues: Distribution and Functions." *Molecular and Cellular Endocrinology* 351 (2): 152–66. https://doi.org/10.1016/j.mce.2012.01.004.

Söderquist, Fanny, Per M. Hellström, and Janet L. Cunningham. 2015. "Human Gastroenteropancreatic Expression of Melatonin and Its Receptors MT1 and MT2." *PLOS ONE* 10 (3): e0120195. https://doi.org/10.1371/journal.pone.0120195.

Solomon, G. D. 1992. "Circadian Rhythms and Migraine." *Cleveland Clinic Journal of Medicine* 59 (3): 326–29.

Song, GiSeon, Kyong-Ah Yoon, HyunYoung Chi, Jaehoon Roh, and Jin-Hee Kim. 2016. "Decreased Concentration of Serum Melatonin in Nighttime Compared with Daytime Female Medical Technologists in South Korea." *Chronobiology International* 33 (9): 1305–10. https://doi.org/10.1080/07420-528.2016.1199562.

Spaeth, Andrea M., David F. Dinges, and Namni Goel. 2015. "Phenotypic Vulnerability of Energy Balance Responses to Sleep Loss in Healthy Adults." *Scientific Reports* 5 (October): 14920. https://doi.org/10.1038/srep14920.

Spiegel, Karine, Rachel Leproult, and Eve Van Cauter. 1999. "Impact of Sleep Debt on Metabolic and Endocrine Function." *Lancet* 354 (9188): 1435–39. https://doi.org/10.1016/S0140-6736(99)01376-8.

Srinivasan, Venkatramanujam, Daniel P. Cardinali, Uddanapalli S. Srinivasan, Charanjit Kaur, Gregory M. Brown, D. Warren Spence, Rüdiger Hardeland, and Seithikurippu R. Pandi-Perumal. 2011. "Therapeutic Potential of Melatonin and Its Analogs in Parkinson's Disease: Focus on Sleep and Neuroprotection." *Therapeutic Advances in Neurological Disorders* 4 (5): 297–317. https://doi.org/10.1177/1756285611406166.

Srinivasan, Venkatramanujam, Edward C. Lauterbach, Khek Yu Ho, Dario Acuna-Castroviejo, Rahimah Zakaria, and Amnon Brzezinski. 2012. "Melatonin in Antinociception: Its Therapeutic Applications." *Current Neuropharmacology* 10 (2): 167–78. http://www.eurekaselect.com/98136/article.

Stankov, B., G. Biella, C. Panara, V. Lucini, S. Capsoni, J. Fauteck, B. Cozzi, and F. Fraschini. 1992. "Melatonin Signal Transduction and Mechanism of Action in the Central Nervous System: Using the Rabbit Cortex as a Model." *Endocrinology* 130 (4): 2152–59. https://doi.org/10.1210/endo.130.4.1312448.

Stankov, B., S. Capsoni, V. Lucini, J. Fauteck, S. Gatti, B. Gridelli, G. Biella, B. Cozzi, and F. Fraschini. 1993. "Autoradiographic Localization of Putative Melatonin Receptors in the Brains of Two Old World Primates: Cercopithecus Aethiops and Papio Ursinus." *Neuroscience* 52 (2): 459–68. https://doi.org/10.1016/0306-4522(93)90172-C.

Stankov, B. M., P. Kolev, Ph. Kumanov, A. Caronno, and J. D. Fauteck. 2010. "Innovation in Dietary Supplement Ingredients: Pharmaceutical Techniques and Body Requirements: Faster Does Not (Always) Mean Better. Time-Defined Controlled Release Is Crucial for Melatonin Efficiency in Primary Sleep Disturbances." *NutraFoods* 13 (3).

Stankov, Bojidar, Bruno Cozzi, Valeria Lucini, Simona Capsoni, Jan Fauteck, Pietro Fumagalli, and Franco Fraschini. 1991. "Localization and Characterization of Melatonin Binding Sites in the Brain of the Rabbit (Oryctolagus Cuniculus) by Autoradiography and in Vitro Ligand-Receptor Binding." *Neuroscience Letters* 133 (1): 68–72. https://doi.org/10.1016/0304-3940(91)90059-3.

Stanley, David A., Sachin S. Talathi, and Paul R. Carney. 2014. "Chronotherapy in the Treatment of Epilepsy." *ChronoPhysiology and Therapy* 2014 (4): 109–23. https://doi.org/10.2147/CPT.S54530.

Stefanovic, Bojana, Natasa Spasojevic, Predrag Jovanovic, Nebojsa Jasnic, Jelena Djordjevic, and Sladjana Dronjak. 2016. "Melatonin Mediated Antidepressant-like Effect in the Hippocampus of Chronic Stress-Induced Depression Rats: Regulating Vesicular Monoamine Transporter 2 and Monoamine Oxidase A Levels." *European Neuropsychopharmacology* 26 (10): 1629–37. https://doi.org/10.1016/j.euroneuro.2016.07.005.

Sundberg, Isak, Mia Ramklint, Mats Stridsberg, Fotios C. Papadopoulos, Lisa Ekselius, and Janet L. Cunningham. 2016. "Salivary Melatonin in Relation to Depressive Symptom Severity in Young Adults." *PLOS ONE* 11 (4): e0152814. https://doi.org/10.1371/journal.pone.0152814.

Tai, Shu-Yu, Shu-Pin Huang, Bo-Ying Bao, and Ming-Tsang Wu. 2016. "Urinary Melatonin-Sulfate/Cortisol Ratio and the Presence of Prostate Cancer: A Case-Control Study." *Scientific Reports* 6 (July): 29606. https://doi.org/10.1038/srep29606.

Tamura, Hiroshi, Akihisa Takasaki, Ichiro Miwa, Ken Taniguchi, Ryo Maekawa, Hiromi Asada, Toshiaki Taketani, et al. 2008. "Oxidative Stress Impairs Oocyte Quality and Melatonin Protects Oocytes from Free Radical Damage and Improves Fertilization Rate." *Journal of Pineal Research* 44 (3): 280–87. https://doi.org/10.1111/j.1600-079X.2007.00524.x.

Tamura, Hiroshi, Akihisa Takasaki, Toshiaki Taketani, Manabu Tanabe, Fumie Kizuka, Lifa Lee, Isao Tamura, et al. 2012. "The Role of Melatonin as an Antioxidant in the Follicle." *Journal of Ovarian Research* 5 (1): 5. https://doi.org/10.1186/1757-2215-5-5.

Tamura, Hiroshi, Yasuhiko Nakamura, Ahmet Korkmaz, Lucien C. Manchester, Dun-Xian Tan, Norihiro Sugino, and Russel J. Reiter. 2009. "Melatonin and the Ovary: Physiological and Pathophysiological Implications." *Fertility and Sterility* 92 (1): 328–43. https://doi.org/10.1016/j.fertnstert.2008.05.016.

Tanev, D., R. Robeva, S. Andonova, V. Decheva, A. Tomova, P. Kumanov, A. Savov, R. Rashkov, and Z. Kolarov. 2016. "Melatonin receptor 1b polymorphisms in women with systemic lupus erythematosus." *Acta Reumatológica Portuguesa* (41): 62–67.

Tang, Yueming, Fabian Preuss, Fred W. Turek, Shriram Jakate, and Ali Keshavarzian. 2009. "Sleep Deprivation Worsens Inflammation and Delays Recovery in a Mouse Model of Colitis." *Sleep Medicine* 10 (6): 597–603. https://doi.org/10.1016/j.sleep.2008.12.009.

Toffol, Elena, Oskari Heikinheimo, and Timo Partonen. 2016. "Biological Rhythms and Fertility: The Hypothalamus–Pituitary– Ovary Axis." *ChronoPhysiology and Therapy* 2016 (6): 15–27. https://doi.org/10.2147/CPT.S84855.

Tosini, Gianluca, Nikita Pozdeyev, Katsuhiko Sakamoto, and P. Michael Iuvone. 2008. "The Circadian Clock System in the Mammalian Retina." *BioEssays* 30 (7): 624–33. https://doi.org/10.1002/bies.20777.

Tosini, Gianluca, P. Michael Iuvone, and Jeffrey H. Boatright. 2013. "Is the Melatonin Receptor Type 1 Involved in the Pathogenesis of Glaucoma?" *Journal of Glaucoma* 22 (July): S49. https://doi.org/10.1097/IJG.0b013e3182934bb4.

Trinder, John, Jan Kleiman, Melinda Carrington, Simon Smith, Sibilah Breen, Nellie Tan, and Young Kim. 2001. "Autonomic Activity during Human Sleep as a Function of Time and Sleep Stage." *Journal of Sleep Research* 10 (4): 253–64. https://doi.org/10.1046/j.1365-2869.2001.00263.x.

Tuomi, Tiinamaija, Cecilia L. F. Nagorny, Pratibha Singh, Hedvig Bennet, Qian Yu, Ida Alenkvist, Bo Isomaa, et al. 2016. "Increased Melatonin Signaling Is a Risk Factor for Type 2 Diabetes." *Cell Metabolism* 23 (6): 1067–77. https://doi.org/10.1016/j.cmet.2016.04.009.

Uchiyama, Makoto, and Steven W. Lockley. 2015. "Non–24-Hour Sleep–Wake Rhythm Disorder in Sighted and Blind Patients." *Sleep Medicine Clinics* 10 (4): 495–516. https://doi.org/10.1016/j.jsmc.2015.07.006.

Valent, Francesca, Marika Mariuz, Giulia Liva, Sara Verri, Sara Arlandini, and Roberto Vivoli. 2016. "Salivary Melatonin and Cortisol and Occupational Injuries among Italian Hospital Workers." *Neurological Sciences* 37 (10): 1613–20. https://doi.org/10.1007/s10072-016-2630-x.

Valenzuela, F. J., J. Vera, C. Venegas, F. Pino, and C. Lagunas. 2015. "Circadian System and Melatonin Hormone: Risk Factors for Complications during

Pregnancy." *Obstetrics and Gynecology International.* https://doi .org/10.1155/2015/825802.

Varoni, Elena Maria, Clelia Soru, Roberta Pluchino, Chiara Intra, and Marcello Iriti. 2016. "The Impact of Melatonin in Research." *Molecules* 21 (2): 240. https://doi.org/10.3390/molecules21020240.

Vaughn, Bradley V., Sean Rotolo, and Heidi L. Roth. 2014. "Circadian Rhythm and Sleep Influences on Digestive Physiology and Disorders." *ChronoPhysiology and Therapy* 2014 (4): 67–77. https://doi.org/10.2147 /CPT.S44806.

Vetter, Céline, Elizabeth E. Devore, Lani R. Wegrzyn, Jennifer Massa, Frank E. Speizer, Ichiro Kawachi, Bernard Rosner, Meir J. Stampfer, and Eva S. Schernhammer. 2016. "Association Between Rotating Night Shift Work and Risk of Coronary Heart Disease Among Women." *JAMA* 315 (16): 1726–34. https://doi.org/10.1001/jama.2016.4454.

Vinther, Anna Gry, and Mogens Helweg Claësson. 2015. "The Influence of Melatonin on the Immune System and Cancer." *Ugeskrift for Laeger* 177 (21): V10140568.

Voiculescu, S.E., N. Zygouropoulos, C.D. Zahiu, and A.M. Zagrean. 2014. "Role of Melatonin in Embryo Fetal Development." *Journal of Medicine and Life* 7 (4): 488–92.

Vriend, Jerry, and Russel J. Reiter. 2014. "Melatonin as a Proteasome Inhibitor. Is There Any Clinical Evidence?" *Life Sciences* 115 (1): 8–14. https://doi.org/10.1016/j.lfs.2014.08.024.

Wadas, Brandon, Jimo Borjigin, Zheping Huang, Jang-Hyun Oh, Cheol-Sang Hwang, and Alexander Varshavsky. 2016. "Degradation of Serotonin N-Acetyltransferase, a Circadian Regulator, by the N-End Rule Pathway." *Journal of Biological Chemistry* 291 (33): 17178–96. https://doi.org/10.1074 /jbc.M116.734640.

Wang, Kun, Yang Wu, Yu Yang, Jie Chen, Danyu Zhang, Yongxin Hu, Zhoujun Liu, et al. 2015. "The Associations of Bedtime, Nocturnal, and Daytime Sleep Duration with Bone Mineral Density in Pre- and Post-Menopausal Women." *Endocrine* 49 (2): 538–48. https://doi.org/10.1007 /s12020-014-0493-6.

Wang, Ri-Xiong, Hui Liu, Li Xu, Hui Zhang, and Rui-Xiang Zhou. 2016. "Melatonin Downregulates Nuclear Receptor RZR/RORγ Expression Causing Growth-Inhibitory and Anti-Angiogenesis Activity in Human Gastric Cancer Cells in Vitro and in Vivo." *Oncology Letters* 12 (2): 897–903. https://doi.org/10.3892/ol.2016.4729.

Watson, Nate, Theo Diamandis, Chiara Gonzales-Portillo, Stephanny Reyes, and Cesar V. Borlongan. 2016. "Melatonin as an Antioxidant for Stroke Neuroprotection." *Cell Transplantation* 25 (5): 883–91. https://doi .org/10.3727/096368915X689749.

Westermann, Jürgen, Tanja Lange, Johannes Textor, and Jan Born. 2015. "System Consolidation During Sleep—A Common Principle Underlying Psychological and Immunological Memory Formation." *Trends in Neurosciences* 38 (10): 585–97. https://doi.org/10.1016/j.tins.2015.07.007.

WHO. Weltgesundheitstag zum ema Diabetes, Diabetes mellitus: Prävention stärken, Versorgung fördern und Surveillance ausbauen." 7 April 2016. Verfügbar unter: https://www.weltgesundheitstag.de/cms/index.asp?inst=wgt-who&snr=11189&t=Dokumentation.

Wong, Patricia M., Brant P. Hasler, Thomas W. Kamarck, Matthew F. Muldoon, and Stephen B. Manuck. 2015. "Social Jetlag, Chronotype, and Cardiometabolic Risk." *Journal of Clinical Endocrinology & Metabolism* 100 (12): 4612–20. https://doi.org/10.1210/jc.2015-2923.

Wu, Anna H., Renwei Wang, Woon-Puay Koh, Frank Z. Stanczyk, Hin-Peng Lee, and Mimi C. Yu. 2008. "Sleep Duration, Melatonin and Breast Cancer among Chinese Women in Singapore." *Carcinogenesis* 29 (6): 1244–48. https://doi.org/10.1093/carcin/bgn100.

Wu, Ying-Hui, Jiang-Ning Zhou, Rawien Balesar, Unga Unmehopa, Aimin Bao, Ralf Jockers, Joop Van Heerikhuize, and Dick F. Swaab. 2006. "Distribution of MT1 Melatonin Receptor Immunoreactivity in the Human Hypothalamus and Pituitary Gland: Colocalization of MT1 with Vasopressin, Oxytocin, and Corticotropin-Releasing Hormone." *Journal of Comparative Neurology* 499 (6): 897–910. https://doi.org/10.1002/cne.21152.

Wulff, Katharina, Derk-Jan Dijk, Benita Middleton, Russell G. Foster, and Eileen M. Joyce. 2012. "Sleep and Circadian Rhythm Disruption in Schizophrenia." *British Journal of Psychiatry* 200 (4): 308–16. https://doi.org/10.1192/bjp.bp.111.096321.

Yan, Shen-Shen, and Wei Wang. 2016. "The Effect of Lens Aging and Cataract Surgery on Circadian Rhythm." *International Journal of Ophthalmology* 9 (7): 1066–74. https://doi.org/10.18240/ijo.2016.07.21.

Yano, Jessica M., Kristie Yu, Gregory P. Donaldson, Gauri G. Shastri, Phoebe Ann, Liang Ma, Cathryn R. Nagler, Rustem F. Ismagilov, Sarkis K. Mazmanian, and Elaine Y. Hsiao. 2015. "Indigenous Bacteria from the Gut Microbiota Regulate Host Serotonin Biosynthesis." *Cell* 161 (2): 264–76. https://doi.org/10.1016/j.cell.2015.02.047.

Yeh, Ta-Chuan, Chin-Bin Yeh, Nian-Sheng Tzeng, and Wei-Chung Mao. 2015. "Adjunctive Treatment with Melatonin Receptor Agonists for Older Delirious Patients with the Sundowning Phenomenon." *Journal of Psychiatry & Neuroscience* 40 (2): E25–26. https://doi.org/10.1503/jpn.140166.

Yildirim, Fatos Belgin, Ozlem Ozsoy, Gamze Tanriover, Yasemin Kaya, Eren Ogut, Burcu Gemici, Sayra Dilmac, Ayse Ozkan, Aysel Agar, and

Mutay Aslan. 2014. "Mechanism of the Beneficial Effect of Melatonin in Experimental Parkinson's Disease." *Neurochemistry International* 79 (December): 1–11. https://doi.org/10.1016/j.neuint.2014.09.005.

Yildirim, Mehmet Erol, Hüseyin Badem, Muzaffer Cakmak, Hakki Yilmaz, Bahadir Kosem, Omer Faruk Karatas, Reyhan Bayrak, and Ersin Cimentepe. 2016. "Melatonin Protects Kidney against Apoptosis Induced by Acute Unilateral Ureteral Obstruction in Rats." *Central European Journal of Urology* 69 (2): 225–30. https://doi.org/10.5173/ceju.2016.770.

Yildirimturk, Senem, Sule Batu, Canan Alatli, Vakur Olgac, Deniz Firat, Yigit Sirin, Senem Yildirimturk, et al. 2016. "The Effects of Supplemental Melatonin Administration on the Healing of Bone Defects in Streptozotocin-Induced Diabetic Rats." *Journal of Applied Oral Science* 24 (3): 239–49. https://doi.org/10.1590/1678-775720150570.

Yonei, Y., A. Hattori, K. Tsutsui, M. Okawa, and B. Ishizuka. 2010. "Effects of Melatonin: Basics Studies and Clinical Applications." *Anti-Aging Medicine* 7 (7): 85–91.

Yu, Hing-Sing, and Russel J. Reiter. 1992. *Melatonin: Biosynthesis, Physiological Effects, and Clinical Applications*. Boca Raton: CRC Press.

Yu, Ji Hee, Chang-Ho Yun, Jae Hee Ahn, Sooyeon Suh, Hyun Joo Cho, Seung Ku Lee, Hye Jin Yoo, et al. 2015. "Evening Chronotype Is Associated with Metabolic Disorders and Body Composition in Middle-Aged Adults." *Journal of Clinical Endocrinology & Metabolism* 100 (4): 1494–1502. https://doi.org/10.1210/jc.2014-3754.

Yuan, Ming, Li-Jing Liu, Ling-Zhi Xu, Tian-You Guo, Xiao-Dong Yue, and Su-Xia Li. 2016. "Effects of Environmental Stress on the Depression-like Behaviors and the Diurnal Rhythm of Corticosterone and Melatonin in Male Rats." *Acta Physiologica Sinica* 68 (3): 215–23.

Zamfir Chiru, A. A., C. R. Popescu, and D. C. Gheorghe. 2014. "Melatonin and Cancer." *Journal of Medicine and Life* 7 (3): 373–74.

Zanette, Simone Azevedo de, Rafael Vercelino, Gabriela Laste, Joanna Ripoll Rozisky, André Schwertner, Caroline Buzzatti Machado, Fernando Xavier, et al. 2014. "Melatonin Analgesia Is Associated with Improvement of the Descending Endogenous Pain-Modulating System in Fibromyalgia: A Phase II, Randomized, Double-Dummy, Controlled Trial." *BMC Pharmacology and Toxicology* 15 (1): 40. https://doi.org/10.1186/2050-6511-15-40.

Zaslavsky, Oleg, Andrea Z. LaCroix, Lauren Hale, Hilary Tindle, and Tamar Shochat. 2015. "Longitudinal Changes in Insomnia Status and Incidence of Physical, Emotional, or Mixed Impairment in Postmenopausal Women Participating in the Women's Health Initiative (WHI) Study." *Sleep Medicine* 16 (3): 364–71. https://doi.org/10.1016/j.sleep.2014.11.008.

Zeng, K., Y. Gao, J. Wan, M. Tong, A. C. Lee, M. Zhao, and Q. Chen. 2016. "The Reduction in Circulating Levels of Melatonin May Be Associated with the Development of Preeclampsia." *Journal of Human Hypertension* 30 (11): 666–71. https://doi.org/10.1038/jhh.2016.37.

Zetner, D., L. P. H. Andersen, and J. Rosenberg. 2016. "Melatonin as Protection Against Radiation Injury: A Systematic Review." *Drug Research* 66 (06): 281–96. https://doi.org/10.1055/s-0035-1569358.

Zhang, S., Y. Qi, H. Zhang, W. He, Q. Zhou, S. Gui, and Y. Wang. 2013. "Melatonin Inhibits Cell Growth and Migration, but Promotes Apoptosis in Gastric Cancer Cell Line, SGC7901." *Biotechnic & Histochemistry* 88 (6): 281–89. https://doi.org/10.3109/10520295.2013.769633.

Ziółko, E., T. Kokot, A. Skubis, B. Sikora, J. Szota-Czyż, C. Kruszniewska-Rajs, J. Wierzgoń, U. Mazurek, E. Grochowska-Niedworok, and M. Muc-Wierzgoń. 2015. "The Profile of Melatonin Receptors Gene Expression and Genes Associated with Their Activity in Colorectal Cancer: A Preliminary Report." *Journal of Biological Regulators and Homeostatic Agents* 29 (4): 823–28.

Additional Sources

Chronobiology.com
www.chronobiology.com

Interchron—A Forum for Chronobiology
www.interchron.org

Picture Verification

Christian Brandst.tter Verlag: Fig. 3, 13, 14, 15, 17, 18
Dr. Jan-Dirk Fauteck: Fig. 2, 4, 5, 6, 7, 8, 9, 10, 11, 12, 16, 19, 20
GettyImages: Fig. 1

About the Authors

Jan-Dirk Fauteck, a chronobiologist, has been a doctor of medicine at the University of Milan and has been researching the role of internal clocks in the human organism for over two decades. He is a founding member of the Academy of Preventive Medicine and Anti-Aging Medicine and is a founding member of the Academy for Preventive Medicine, "ea3m." He is also a founding member and secretary of Interchron, the international forum for chronobiology.

Dr. Andrea Eder, holds a PhD specializing in comparative literature and German language from the University of Vienna. She has spent many years as a lecturer and editor in publishing, in online and print media, for academic organizations, public administration, and companies in various industries.

Foreword Contributor:

Russel J. Reiter, PhD, Dr. h.c. mult., is a professor of cell biology at the University of Texas and has been researching melatonin for more than fifty years. He has more than one thousand original works on the topic of melatonin and is the most cited author when it comes to melatonin.